W9-AEV-055

DISCARDED

ANNUAL REVIEW OF NURSING RESEARCH

Volume 12, 1994

EDITORS

Joyce J. Fitzpatrick, Ph.D.
Dean and Professor
Frances Payne Bolton School
   of Nursing
Case Western Reserve University
Cleveland, Ohio

Joanne S. Stevenson, Ph.D.
Professor
College of Nursing
The Ohio State University
Columbus, Ohio

ASSOCIATE EDITOR

Nikki S. Polis, Ph.D.
Researcher
Frances Payne Bolton School
   of Nursing
Case Western Reserve University
Cleveland, Ohio

ADVISORY BOARD

Violet Barkauskas, Ph.D.
School of Nursing
University of Michigan
Ann Arbor, Michigan

Marie Cowan, Ph.D.
School of Nursing
University of Washington
Seattle, Washington

Claire Fagin, Ph.D.
School of Nursing
University of Pennsylvania
Philadelphia, Pennsylvania

Suzanne Feetham, Ph.D.
National Institute for Nursing
   Research
National Institutes of Health
Bethesda, Maryland

Phyllis Giovannetti, Sc.D.
Faculty of Nursing
University of Alberta
Edmonton, Alberta, Canada

Ada Sue Hinshaw, Ph.D.
National Institute for Nursing
   Research
National Institutes of Health
Bethesda, Maryland

Kathleen McCormick, Ph.D.
Office of the Forum for Quality
   and Effectiveness in Health Care
Agency for Health Care Policy and
   Research
Rockville, Maryland

Jane Norbeck, D.N.Sc.
School of Nursing
University of California,
   San Francisco
San Francisco, California

Christine Tanner, Ph.D.
School of Nursing
Oregon Health Sciences University
Portland, Oregon

Roma Lee Taunton, Ph.D.
School of Nursing
The University of Kansas
Kansas City, Kansas

Harriet Werley, Ph.D.
School of Nursing
University of Wisconsin-Milwaukee
Milwaukee, Wisconsin
Founding Editor
*Annual Review of Nursing
   Research*

ANNUAL REVIEW OF NURSING RESEARCH

Volume 12, 1994

Joyce J. Fitzpatrick, Ph.D.
Joanne S. Stevenson, Ph.D.

Editors

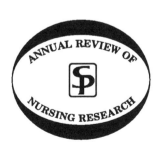

SPRINGER PUBLISHING COMPANY
New York

CARL A. RUDISILL LIBRARY
LENOIR-RHYNE COLLEGE

RT
81.5
. A55
V 12
aug. 1994

Order ANNUAL REVIEW OF NURSING RESEARCH. Volume 12, 1994, prior to publication and receive a 10% discount. An order coupon can be found at the back of this volume.

Copyright © 1994 by Springer Publishing Company. Inc.
All rights reserved

No part of this publication may be reproduced, stored in a retrieval system, or transmitted in any form or by any means, electronic, mechanical, photocopying, recording, or otherwise, without the prior permission of Springer Publishing Company, Inc.

Springer Publishing Company, Inc.
536 Broadway
New York, NY 10012

94 95 96 97 98 / 5 4 3 2 1

ISBN-0-8261 8231-3
ISSN-0739-6686

ANNUAL REVIEW OF NURSING RESEARCH is indexed in *Cumulative Index to Nursing and Allied Health Literature and Index Medicus.*

Printed in the United States of America

Contents

Preface

This is the twelfth volume of the *Annual Review of Nursing Research* (*ARNR*) series, which began in 1983. As introduced in Volume 11, the beginning of the book's second decade, our goal is to select chapter topics that are more specific in focus.

Part I, Research on Nursing Practice, follows the theme of significant clinical issues. In Chapter 1, Nancy M. Ryan-Wenger presents research on psychogenic pain in children. Chapter 2 includes discussion of fatigue during the childbearing period by Renée A. Milligan and Linda C. Pugh. Terry Fulmer reviews the research on elder mistreatment in Chapter 3, and Clarann Weinert and Mary E. Burman review research on rural health and health-seeking behaviors in Chapter 4.

Research on Nursing Care Delivery is the focus of Part II. In Chapter 5, Sandra R. Edwardson and Phyllis B. Giovannetti review research on nursing workload measurement systems. A review of hospice nursing as symptom control is presented by Inge B. Corless. Part III, which focuses on Nursing Education Research, includes one chapter, a review of registered nurses and the baccalaureate degree by Mary Beth Mathews and Lucille L. Travis. Part IV, Research on the Profession of Nursing, also includes one chapter, a review of research on minorities in nursing by Diana L. Morris and May L. Wykle.

Part V has served as a category for chapters that do not easily fit the content theme of Part I or the categories included in the other components. Part V also has included chapters regarding nursing research in other countries. In this twelfth volume, Part V includes a chapter on Native American health by Sharol F. Jacobson and a chapter on nursing research in Korea by Elizabeth C. Choi.

Our thanks are extended to the new Advisory Board members who joined us as of Volume 11: Violet Barkauskas, Marie Cowan, Claire Fagin, Suzanne Feetham, Phyllis Giovannetti, Ada Sue Hinshaw, Kathleen McCormick, Jane Norbeck, Christine Tanner, Roma Lee Taunton, and Harriet Werley. Our Advisory Board members play a major role in setting directions for the future, as well as recommending authors, chapters, and reviewers for each volume.

We look forward to your continuing involvement in this important series. We continue to welcome suggestions for topics, authors, and expert reviewers, as well as your suggestions about how we can improve this *ARNR* series. Please let us know your ideas.

JOYCE J. FITZPATRICK
SENIOR EDITOR

Contributors

Mary E. Burman, Ph.D.
School of Nursing
University of Wyoming
Laramie, WY

Elizabeth C. Choi, Ph.D.
School of Nursing
George Mason University
Fairfax, Virginia

Inge B. Corless, Ph.D.
Graduate Program in Nursing
MGH Institute of Health Professions
Boston, Massachusetts

Sandra R. Edwardson, Ph.D.
School of Nursing
University of Minnesota
Minneapolis, Minnesota

Terry T. Fulmer, Ph.D.
School of Nursing
Columbia University
New York, New York

Phyllis B. Giovannetti, Sc.D.
Faculty of Nursing
University of Alberta
Edmonton, Alberta, Canada

Sharol F. Jacobson, Ph.D.
College of Nursing
University of Oklahoma Health
    Sciences Center
Oklahoma City, Oklahoma

Mary Beth Mathews, Ph.D.
Nursing Education, Development,
    and Research
Riverside Methodist Hospitals
Columbus, Ohio

Renée A. Milligan, Ph.D.
School of Nursing
Georgetown University
Washington, D.C.

Diana L. Morris, Ph.D.
Frances Payne Bolton School of
    Nursing
Case Western Reserve University
Cleveland, Ohio

Linda C. Pugh, Ph.D.
School of Nursing
The Johns Hopkins University
Baltimore, Maryland

Nancy M. Ryan-Wenger, Ph.D.
College of Nursing
The Ohio State University
Columbus, Ohio

Lucille L. Travis, Ph.D.
Frances Payne Bolton School of
  Nursing
Case Western Reserve University
Cleveland, Ohio

May L. Wykle, Ph.D.
Frances Payne Bolton School of
  Nursing
Case Western Reserve University
Cleveland, Ohio

Clarann Weinert, S.C., Ph.D.
College of Nursing
Montana State University
Bozeman, MT

FORTHCOMING

ANNUAL REVIEW OF
NURSING RESEARCH, Volume 13

Tentative Contents

PART I
Research on Nursing Practice

Chapter 1

Psychogenic Pain in Children

NANCY M. RYAN-WENGER
COLLEGE OF NURSING
THE OHIO STATE UNIVERSITY

CONTENTS

The literature generally differentiates psychogenic pain from malingering, organic pain, and dysfunctional pain. *Malingering* (e.g., feigned abdominal pain) is rarely observed during childhood (Li, 1987). Some abdominal pain is labelled *organic* if the pain originates from and is manifested as a disease or disorder in a specific body organ or site, such as ulcerative colitis (Coleman, 1992). In the case of organic pain, there is a specific medical or surgical diagnosis. Pain is labelled *dysfunctional* when it is caused by normal variations in physiological processes (e.g., stool retention). Psychogenic pain, such as recurrent abdominal pain, is often labelled as such when pain is periodic in nature, the child is otherwise healthy in appearance, no specific medical or surgical diagnosis or dysfunction is apparent, and a "psychological" origin is suspected. The most popular (but relatively untested) theory is that psychogenic pain originates from a primary psychologic response to endogenous or exogenous stressors. A secondary physiologic stress response is manifested as pain at a variety of organ sites (Coleman, 1992). The theory does not specify the exact biological mechanism that elicits pain, however. Several terms are used to describe the same phenomenon, including psychogenic, psychosomatic, functional, recurrent, periodic, and nonspecific. For consistency, the term "psychogenic" is used in this review. Four sites of psychogenic pain in children are commonly referred to in the literature: abdominal pain, limb pain, headache, and chest pain.

DEFINITION OF TERMS

Abdominal Pain

Most clinicians and researchers have used Apley and Naish's (1958) original criteria for the diagnosis of psychogenic recurrent abdominal pain (RAP): pains at least once per month for 3 consecutive months, severe enough to limit activities, and intermittent asymptomatic periods. Pain is typically periumbilical, and concomitant autonomic symptoms such as nausea, perspiration, palpitations, and flushing or pallor are common. RAP occurs in 10% to 15% of all children, primarily during the school-age period, and more often in girls than boys (Li, 1987; Poole, 1984).

Limb Pain

Limb pains often have been erroneously referred to as "growing pains" because they tend to disappear when the child stops growing; however, the pains are not related to the growth process. Limb pain presents as deep, intermittent pain in the muscles of both calves or thighs (Szer, 1989), and is not associated with limping or limited mobility (Peterson, 1986). Naish and Apley (1951) developed criteria for psychogenic limb pain which included: a three-month history of pain, intermittent symptom-free intervals, occurs late in the day or awakens the child at night, and is severe enough to limit activity. Limb pain occurs in about 4.2% (Szer, 1989) to 15% (Schechter, 1984) of all children, primarily during the school-age period, and in girls more often than boys (Peterson, 1986).

Headache

Muscle contraction headaches of psychogenic origin typically occur daily and build in intensity during the day. The pain has been described as an ache or simply as something that "hurts," usually in the frontal area (Barlow, 1984). There has been much disagreement about the prevalence of psychogenic headaches in children, ranging from 5% to 20% of children (Barlow, 1984; Chu & Shinnar, 1992; Gascon, 1984; Passchier & Orlebeke, 1985; Schechter, 1984). There also has been disagreement about the percentage of headaches that are psychogenic in origin. Psychogenic headaches have been noted more often in adolescents than in younger children, and more often in girls than boys (Choquet & Menke, 1987; Sillanpää, 1983a, 1983b).

Chest Pain

Recurrent chest pain has not been well described in terms of specific location, intensity, or frequency, but has been reported to account for 650,000 physician visits annually in 10- to 21-year-olds (Coleman, 1984). In a study of urban black adolescents, chest pain was the seventh most common presenting symptom (Brunswick, Boyle, & Tarica, 1979). Chest pain has been reported in adolescents more often than younger children (Coleman, 1984), and in boys more often than girls (Selbst, 1985).

ORGANIZATION OF THE REVIEW

A critical analysis and overview of the corpus of published research on psychogenic pain in children is provided, followed by a synthesis of the research on 12 major variables related to psychogenic pain. When available, a description of the stated or implied underlying theoretical framework or hypotheses precedes the discussion of empirical work on each variable. Findings for which there is consensus, disparity, and/or equivocation are presented. Each subsection ends with a critical review of related intervention research and suggestions for further research.

The literature for this review was obtained from computerized literature searches, hand searches from medical, nursing, and social science indexes, and references from published research. The empirical work included in this review was limited to all data-based research on the four common types of psychogenic pain in children, published from January 1980 to September 1992 ($N = 66$).

OVERVIEW OF THE RESEARCH

Research on psychogenic pain in children was conducted by scientists from numerous disciplines, including medicine (32), psychiatry (14), psychology (13), nursing (1), and other health-related disciplines (6). The scientists from behavioral science disciplines focus mainly on psychogenic or environmental and familial factors, whereas behavioral scientists focus primarily on physical or organic mechanisms to explain the pain. Studies have been conducted in numerous geographic areas including the United States (27), Western Europe (15), Great Britain (11), Canada (9), and Australia (4); it is apparent that psychogenic pain in children is a concern for children in most First World countries.

Samples of children with psychogenic pain were derived primarily from outpatient clinics and pediatrician offices (45), but also from schools or community groups (13), hospitals (5), and the emergency department (1). The source of subjects was not clearly stated in two studies. There is some argument about the equivalence of samples drawn from schools, clinics, and hospitals. The characteristics of school children with psychogenic symptoms who are *not* seen in the health care system may be different from children whose parents seek medical intervention for them through clinics, and may differ also from children whose parents are not satisfied with a psychogenic diagnosis even after hospitalization or unnecessary surgery (Hughes, 1984). Disparate results among these studies did not appear to be a function of the type of sample used thus it was possible to integrate the findings from all the studies.

Regarding research design, of the 66 studies, 61% (40) were comparative studies and 39% (26) were single-sample designs, 15 of which were descriptive studies, and 11 of which were studies of treatment interventions. Only one of the intervention studies was not controlled; half the studies employed an experimental and control-group design, whereas in the other half of the studies, subjects served as their own controls.

Of the 40 comparative studies, children with psychogenic pain were compared with both healthy and "sick" children (17), with healthy children only (10), or with "sick" children only (13). Sick children included those who had organic illnesses with symptoms similar to the psychogenic symptoms (22), chronic illnesses (8), unrelated acute illnesses (3), behavioral disorders (6) and psychiatric illnesses (1). One researcher compared children with adults. The rationale for selection of these comparative groups was rarely given; therefore the utility of the findings for practice is unclear. Samples of healthy or asymptomatic children in the comparative studies were obtained from schools or the community (16), from children seen for routine well-child physical examinations in clinics (9) and from previously published literature (2).

All the investigators used convenience samples and subjects were sometimes deliberately selected because of specific characteristics. None of the research reports included a power analysis or rationale for the sample size selected. Although the number of subjects in single sample descriptive studies ranged from 16 to 2,921, over half the studies had more than 100 subjects. The intervention studies had from 1 to 106 subjects per group, whereas the comparative descriptive studies had from 1 to 539 subjects per group. Cohen's (1977) sample size guidelines were applied to the 51 comparative and intervention studies, with alpha set at 0.05 and power at 0.80. If a moderate effect size was predicted, only five studies would have had a sufficient sample size. If a large effect size was predicted, 26 studies would have had a sufficient sample size; however, a large effect size may not be justifiable.

Psychometrically sound instruments appropriate for children were used in the majority of studies, and appropriate statistical procedures were used to analyze the data. Most of the findings were based primarily on descriptive statistics, nonparametric, and simple inferential statistics such as t-tests and analysis of variance, and only a few authors identified an alpha level of significance a priori. Despite the inevitable limitations of individual studies, similarities among the findings suggested that the phenomenon observed was fairly robust; therefore, some conclusions can be drawn from a group of studies. To avoid the use of numerous p-values in the discussion of specific studies, the term "significant" is used throughout this review to reflect findings with p-values at 0.05 or better.

In general, there were two positions taken by investigators of psychogenic pain in children. Those who supported the notion of psychogenic origin of pain primarily studied family, environmental, and psychosocial variables, whereas nonsupporters (i.e., those who supported some biologic cause) primarily studied biophysical variables as alternative etiologies for the pain.

INCIDENCE AND IMPACT OF PSYCHOGENIC PAIN IN CHILDREN

An estimated 10% to 15% of all children experience psychogenic headache, abdominal, chest, or limb pain (Apley, 1975; Poole, 1984). The actual incidence and prevalence of psychogenic pain in children is not known because inconsistent criteria have been used for the term "psychogenic," however. Some researchers relied on physician diagnoses, whereas other researchers included any child with parent-, teacher- or self-report of frequent pain symptoms. Further, the operationalization of the term "frequent" has varied from two episodes per week to one or more episodes per year. Many researchers did not require physician verification of psychogenicity based on the wide belief that only 5% of children with such pain symptoms have a medical or surgical diagnosis (Jay & Tomasi, 1981; Li, 1987; Poole, 1984).

The morbidity of psychogenic pain in children was reflected in school absenteeism, frequent and expensive physician visits, and poor long-term prognoses. Children with psychogenic symptoms missed more school days than asymptomatic children (Crossley, 1982; Hodges, Kline, Barbero, & Woodruff, 1985b; Robinson, Alverez, & Dodge, 1989; Wasserman, Whitington, & Rivara, 1988), as many as 26 to 30 days per school year (Bury, 1987; Hodges et al., 1985). Stomachaches and headaches accounted for 25% (Nader & Brink, 1981) and 41% (Stephenson, 1983) of all visits to the offices of school nurses in two different elementary schools. In a self-initiated school health clinic, 15% of the children made over half of all the visits with a variety of complaints, the most common of which were stomach aches and headaches (Lewis, Lewis, Lorrimer, & Palmer, 1977).

Over a 6–year period, 17.3% of the children's services provided by a health maintenance organization were for psychogenic symptoms (Starfield et al., 1980) and more than 20% of those children had at least eight additional acute and nonacute problems (Starfield et al., 1984). Complaints of abdominal pain accounted for 3% (n = 371) of all emergency department visits during 4 seasonally diverse months (Reynolds & Jaffe, 1990). Based on urine and hematologic laboratory results, chest x-rays, barium enemas, careful histories, and physical examinations, 64.4% were classified as medical diagnoses, 6.5% as surgical diagnoses, and 29.1% as "nonspecific" or psychogenic. From a sample of all 6–year old children in a new industrial town in Great Britain (n = 494), 34% experienced more than three episodes of abdominal pain within the past 3 months, according to parent report. Although 58% of those children had been seen by a general practitioner, no specific diagnosis or treatment was offered and parents reported the physician visit as "unhelpful" (Faull & Nicol, 1986). The cost of a typical 3–day outpatient and inpatient medical evaluation of a child with RAP was estimated to be $3060 per child in 1986 (Li, 1987). Such costs are disproportional to the percentage of children (about 5%) for whom a specific medical or surgical diagnosis for frequent headache, abdominal, chest or limb pain typically is found.

Stress research has shown that exaggerated and prolonged somatic responses to stress may result in structural changes and tissue damage (Eaton, Peterson, & Davies, 1981; Henker, 1984). This prolonged response may be responsible for the fact that children do not necessarily "grow out" of these symptoms. Longitudinal and retrospective studies have shown that RAP is still present in 64% of a sample of children after 3 months (Crossley, 1982), in 68% after an average of 9 months (Wasserman et al., 1988), and 66% after 1 to 7 years (Bury, 1987). About one-fourth of school-age children who originally had RAP reportedly developed *other* pains several years later (Crossley, 1982; Magni, Pierri, & Donzelli, 1987). After 12 years, one-half of the most frequent visitors to the self-initiated school clinic still complained of stomachaches and headaches as adults (Lewis & Lewis, 1989). One 20–year follow-up study revealed that migraines were now a problem for a large percentage of adults who had RAP (70%), limb pain (66%) and headaches (33%) when they were children (Salmon, 1985).

FAMILY AND ENVIRONMENTAL VARIABLES

Family Functioning

Some dysfunctional family systems maintain their equilibrium only as long as a family member has a somatic symptom that serves to deflect attention from factors that would ordinarily result in conflict, for example, marital, financial, or substance abuse problems (Haggerty, 1983; Wood et al., 1989). Using ancecdotal situations to describe the "psychosomatic family mode," Castleberry (1988) demonstrated how the power of "family rules" in dysfunctional families fosters and maintains psychogenic symptoms in children. The secondary gain for the child is increased attention and school avoidance. Most research findings do not support the hypothesis that children with psychogenic pain come from dysfunctional families, however.

When psychometrically sound measures were used, four studies with clinical or school samples showed no significant differences in family functioning between asymptomatic children and children with RAP (Raymer, Weininger, & Hamilton, 1984; Robinson, Greene, & Walker, 1988; Sawyer, Davidson, Goodwin, & Crettenden, 1987; Wasserman et al., 1988), chest pain and limb pain (Robinson et al., 1988). In a study in which family functioning was measured by observation rather than self-report, Castleberry's psychosomatic family model was supported (Wood et al., 1989). Videotapes of family interactions revealed that families of children with RAP demonstrated enmeshment, rigidity, and poor conflict resolution, but not overprotection, as expected. The authors postulated that the child with RAP serves as a scapegoat for family conflict. Interrater reliability of interaction scores between two independent observers was 0.70–0.90. No comparison of families with asymptomatic children was made, however, to determine if similar family interaction styles exist.

Results are equivocal on the prevalence of marital problems and/or single-parent families with respect to psychogenic symptoms in children. In one study of children with chest pain (n = 100, 91% black), there were more frequent family separations than the national statistics would have predicted (Pantell & Goodman, 1983). Other researchers have shown that single-parent families were significantly more prevalent in samples of children with RAP compared to samples of asymptomatic children (30% versus 18.6%) (Crossley, 1982). Similar findings are available for children with headaches (39% versus 9%) (Larsson, 1988). On the other hand, four studies with samples of fewer than 50 subjects per group found no differences in parental marital status (Faull & Nicol, 1986; McGrath, Goodman, Firestone, Shipman, & Peters, 1983; Walker & Greene, 1989; Zuckerman, Stevenson, & Bailey, 1987).

The weak empirical support for the theory linking family functioning with psychogenic pain can be interpreted in many ways: the theory is incorrect, the operational definitions of family functioning are not sufficiently sensitive, or other methodological problems have clouded the relationship. Further, the role of family functioning in the etiology of symptoms cannot be evaluated without prospective studies. A more in-depth theoretical analysis of the connection between family systems and psychogenic symptoms is needed before further descriptive research is done.

Family History of Pain

Investigators have clearly shown that a family history of chronic pain or other symptoms was more typical of children with psychogenic pain than asymptomatic children (Burg, 1987; Wasserman et al., 1988; Mortimer & Good, 1990; Larsson, 1988; Pantell & Goodman, 1983; Garber, Zeman, & Walker, 1990). There were three potential explanations for the appearance of symptoms in children belonging to these families (Apley, 1975). Children may have an inherited predisposition for symptoms similar to their parents' symptoms; children may learn symptom-behavior from observation of their parents; or, parents' fussing over children's somatic complaints, while ignoring other behavior (e.g., aggression) may serve to reinforce the use of symptoms for attention (Apley, 1975). A fourth explanation may be that children have the same undiagnosed medical or surgical "organic" problem as their parents.

Compared to family members of asymptomatic children, more family members of children with RAP had a history of RAP themselves (Bury, 1987), peptic ulcer (Wasserman et al., 1988), unexplained pain (Geist, 1989; Magni, Pierri, & Donzelli, 1987), migraines and "nervous trouble" (Mortimer & Good, 1990; Robinson et al., 1989), depression, anxiety, and somatization disorders (Walker & Greene, 1989), and lengthy parental illness over the past 3 months to 1 year (Crossley, 1982; Garber et al., 1990; Zuckerman, Stevenson, & Bailey, 1987). Similarly, 40% of children with headaches had parents with a history of headaches (Larsson, 1988; Werder & Sargent, 1984), and parents of 45%

of children with chest pain also had chest-related problems (Pantell & Goodman, 1983). In studies that differentiated among family members, typically, mothers rather than fathers had the majority of symptoms (Garber et al., 1990; Mortimer & Good, 1990; Robinson et al., 1989; Routh & Ernst, 1984; Walker & Greene, 1989). Only two research teams showed no difference in family history of pain between RAP and asymptomatic children (Faull & Nicol, 1986; McGrath et al., 1983). Although there has been ample descriptive work, theory-generating and theory-testing research is needed to explain whether children have psychogenic pain because the pains are inherited, learned, or reinforced.

Stressful Life Events

Two distinct theories regarding the relationship between stressful life events and illness have been tested with children who have psychogenic pain. One theory hypothesizes that the amount of life change caused by stressful life events, not the events per se, puts an individual at risk for health problems (Holmes & Masuda, 1974). Six research teams used life change unit (LCU) measures of stress, but none of the six studies had a large enough sample ($n =$ 16 to 31 per group) to detect a moderate effect size. Data from four of the six studies revealed no significant differences between children with RAP or headaches and asymptomatic children (Kowal & Pritchard, 1990; McGrath et al., 1983; Raymer et al., 1984; Wasserman et al., 1988). The hypothesis was supported by two studies of children with RAP who had significantly higher LCU scores than asymptomatic children (Hodges, Kline, Barbero, & Flanery, 1984; Robinson et al., 1989). Item analysis of life events in one of the studies showed that children with RAP experienced more health- and death-related stressors than asymptomatic children (p-value not reported) (Hodges et al., 1984). A step-wise multiple regression showed that the LCU score explained 10% of the variance and was a significant predictor of the severity of headache pain in 23 children (Kowal & Pritchard, 1990). The validity of this line of research is compromised by the fact that data in four of the five LCU studies were collected from parents rather than from the children themselves. Further, in each instrument used, the amount of life change assigned to each event was determined by adults without validation by children (Ryan, 1988).

An alternative theory is that the individual's own appraisal of a stressful life event as a threat, benign/positive, or a challenge is one determinant of the outcome of the stress-coping process (Lazarus, 1966, 1991). Self-report methods in which stress was measured from the children's perspective were used in five studies. Data from all of the studies indicated that children with RAP (Adams & Weaver, 1986; Greene, Walker, Hickson, & Thompson, 1985; Robinson, Greene, & Walker, 1988; Sharrer & Ryan-Wenger, 1991), headache

(Adams & Weaver, 1986; Larsson, 1988), limb pain (Robinson et al., 1988), and chest pain (Adams & Weaver, 1986) had significantly higher stress scores than asymptomatic children. Sample sizes ranged from 12 to 70 per group. In the study with the largest sample size, an investigator-designed an 11–item measure with no established reliability and validity was used (Larsson, 1988), whereas previously tested instruments were used in the other four studies. In a single sample study, 100 children with chest pain were interviewed regarding the incidence of negative life events prior to the onset of chest pain (Pantell & Goodman, 1983); however, the reliability of interview data was not established. It was noted that 26% and 31% of the children identified negative life events in the previous 3 and 6 months, respectively, but there was no comparison group of asymptomatic children to determine the extent to which these percentages are abnormal. When asked what they think caused their own headaches, 30% of 198 elementary and 40% of 660 secondary school children named "stress" as the cause (Passchier & Orlebeke, 1985). In the same study, a stepwise multiple regression revealed that self-identified fear of failure and school problems each contributed a significant proportion of the variance in the frequency, intensity, duration, degree of interference with normal activity, and consequences of headache pain.

In all but two of the above studies (Pantell & Goodman, 1983; Robinson et al., 1989), researchers examined stressful life events without regard to the timing of the event compared to the symptom. More research is needed to determine the extent to which stressful events are precipitant to or concomitant with the symptom. It may be that the experience of pain is unrelated to stress, but that the pain heightens one's perceptions of stress. Clinical intervention research is needed in which children with psychogenic pain are helped to identify and modify their own stressors and to cope with stressors that cannot be changed. This type of research will further test the hypothetical links between stressful life events and psychogenic pain in children.

PSYCHOSOCIAL VARIABLES

Depression, Anxiety, and Self-Esteem

There is no specific theory that links psychogenic pain in children with depression, anxiety, or self-esteem, but most research on the relationship among these variables was conducted to test the clinical observation that these children appear to have emotional problems and lack self-esteem. Research findings are divided on the issue of depression and psychogenic pain. Significant positive correlations ($r = 0.17$–0.48) between depression and somatic symptom scores were observed for children with RAP, headache, and limb pain (Larsson, 1991). When criteria from the Diagnostic and Statistical Manual of Mental Disorders,

Version III (DSM-III; American Psychiatric Association, 1980) were applied, 5 out of 13 children with RAP were diagnosed with a major depressive disorder, as opposed to none of the 16 asymptomatic children in the study (no *p*-value reported) (Garber et al., 1990). Significantly higher depression rating scales scores were found by self-report for children with RAP (*n* = 41) (Walker & Greene, 1989) and by parent-report for children with headaches (*n* = 70) (Larsson, 1988). Conflicting outcomes occurred in four studies that compared small groups of children with RAP or headaches (*n* = 16 to 30) to asymptomatic children. The investigators found no significant differences in depression scale scores (Kowal & Pritchard, 1990; McGrath et al., 1983; Raymer et al., 1984; Routh & Ernst, 1984). Investigators used reliable and valid depression inventories appropriate for children in each of these studies.

The preponderance of evidence indicated that children with psychogenic pain tend to be anxious. Scores on an investigator-developed Habitual Somatic Discomfort Questionnaire (HSDQ) correlated positively with anxiety scores for 90 13– to 18–year old children (*r* = 0.30–0.42), but not for 11-year old children (Rauste-von Wright & von Wright, 1981). In another study, a stepwise multiple regression showed that for 23 children with headaches, anxiety scores explained 22.4% of the variance and was a significant predictor of the severity of headache pain (Kowal & Pritchard, 1990). A single sample study showed that 21 out of 22 children with RAP met DSM-III criteria for several anxiety disorders (Astrada, Licamele, Walsh, & Kessler, 1981). Through a clinical interview, one researcher found that 84% of clinic RAP patients worried about themselves and their parents, which is more than twice that expected of the general population of children (Wasserman et al., 1988). Clinical interviews with children with RAP resulted in significantly more DSM-III diagnoses of "over-anxious disorder" compared to asymptomatic children in two studies (Garber et al., 1990; Hodges et al., 1985a). Similarly, when reliable and valid self-report instruments were used, anxiety scores of children with RAP (Hodges et al., 1985b; Walker & Greene, 1989) and headache (Larsson, 1988) were significantly higher than scores of asymptomatic children. With respect to long-term prognosis, a retrospective chart review indicated that for 17% of the sample, RAP in childhood was a precursor to somatization disorder (hysteria) in adults (Ernst, Routh, & Harper, 1984).

In three of the above studies, mothers of children with RAP also had significantly higher anxiety scores than mothers of asymptomatic children (Garber et al., 1990; Hodges et al., 1985b; Walker & Greene, 1989). Results are equivocal, however, for the fathers of children with RAP, that is, their anxiety scores were significantly higher in one study (Hodges et al., 1985b), but nonsignificant in another study (Garber et al., 1990). One study revealed no differences in anxiety scores between asymptomatic children and 10 children with RAP; however, anxiety scores were based on the children's response to one question, "How nervous are you?" on a scale of 1 to 10 (Feuerstein, Barr, Francoeur, Houle, & Rafman, 1982). Similarly, no differences between children with headache and asymptomatic children ($n = 23$ per group) were found when a psychometrically sound measure was used (Kowal & Pritchard, 1990).

Data from three studies showed that despite small sample sizes ($n = 16$ to 31), self-esteem scores of children with headache, RAP, limb, or chest pain were signficantly lower than scores of asymptomatic (Raymer et al., 1984; Robinson et al., 1988) or chronically ill children (Adams & Weaver, 1986). One-third of the 16 children with RAP had scores more than 2 SD below the mean on the Coopersmith Self-Esteem Inventory (Raymer et al., 1984). A six-item measure of self-esteem, with no evidence of reliability or validity, was used in one of the above studies (Robinson et al., 1988).

Because all the above studies were conducted at one point in time, when children had already developed symptoms, the above findings only support clinical observations that children with psychogenic pain tend to be depressed, anxious, or have low self-esteem; there are no prospective studies which indicate that these variables are *etiological*. The major gap in this line of research is the lack of a theoretical base for linking psychogenic pain with depression, anxiety, or self-esteem. Without a viable theory to describe, explain, and predict relationships among these variables, further descriptive work of this type does not build knowledge about psychogenic pain in children, hence both prevention and intervention studies would be premature.

Problem Behavior

Research results supported clinical observations that children who experience psychogenic pain often demonstrate problem behavior at home. Using the Child Behavior Checklist (CBCL), a popular psychometric measure, several researchers found significantly more problem behavior in children with RAP ($n = 13$ to 41) compared to asymptomatic children (Garber et al., 1990; Sawyer et al., 1987; Walker & Greene, 1989; Wasserman et al., 1988). Similarly, structured interviews with parents revealed that children with RAP and headache were significantly more dependent and/or had more fears (Zuckerman et al., 1987), were more "neurotic" (Crossley, 1982), and displayed more antisocial behavior (Faull & Nicol, 1986) than asymptomatic children. Only one parental interview study showed no difference between symptomatic and asymptomatic groups on problem behavior at home (Davison, Faull, & Nicol, 1986). It is possible that psychogenic pain makes children irritable, causing them to act out their distress. On the other hand, parental responses may have been biased.

Contrary to home behavior, school behavior as reported by teachers on the CBCL (Garber et al., 1990; Walker & Greene, 1989; Wasserman et al., 1988) or structured interview (Crossley, 1982), did not differ among children with and without psychogenic pain except in one study in which children with RAP displayed more fidgeting, humming, and failure to complete work than asymptomatic children (Faull & Nicol, 1986).

There are several possible explanations for the differences observed between school and home behavior: the differences may be real; either parents' or teachers' perceptions may be inaccurate or biased; or, the family environment may foster problem behavior, whereas the school environment may not foster or tolerate it. Whether problem behavior is a cause or effect of psychogenic pain in children has not been established by these cross-sectional studies, nor is there a theory that links these two variables. A careful theoretical analysis is needed before further research of this type is conducted.

Coping Strategies

There are clear theoretical links between psychogenic pain and the stress-coping process. Lazarus and Launier (1978) emphasized that the frequency and severity of stressors may be less important to an individual's physical, psychological, and emotional health than the effectiveness of coping strategies. Patterns of coping develop during childhood and often are carried into adulthood (Garmezy & Rutter, 1983). Mechanic (1983) suggested that the increased introspection and self-awareness that accompanies adolescent development results in increased psychological pain and symptom reporting, whereas successful coping strategies help to decrease such responses.

Although coping behavior is an integral part of the stress process, it has rarely been studied with regard to psychogenic pain. In one study of coping strategies used by a small sample of school children ($n = 25$) with and without RAP, there were no differences in mean coping frequency or effectiveness scores (Sharrer & Ryan-Wenger, 1991). Mean scores on coping measures may be less informative than an examination of *specific* coping strategies that children use to deal with stressors, however. In one study, headache intensity was associated with use of more passive coping strategies and less use of social support according to the Dutch Coping Questionnaire (van den Bree, Passchier, & Emmen, 1990). On the other hand, children with RAP used significantly more isolating and social support strategies, whereas children without RAP used distraction, relaxation, and cognitive strategies significantly more often, as shown on the Schoolagers' Coping Strategies Inventory (Sharrer & Ryan-Wenger, 1991).

In an intervention study at a 3-month follow-up, seven (87.5%) of eight children with RAP were pain-free after an 8-week cognitive coping skills training program, compared to 37.5% of the children in the wait-list control group (Sanders et al., 1989). The intervention included self-monitoring, self-instruction, self-efficacy statements, relaxation, self-administration of rewards, and imagery techniques. The extent to which children continue to use these techniques beyond the training program is difficult to monitor and therefore, it is difficult to attribute long-term change to the intervention. There have been several studies of relaxation protocols as interventions (discussed under "Muscle Tension"), but in these studies, relaxation was used for symptom-management, not as a strategy to manage stress per se.

In summary, the variable of problem behavior lacks a theoretical basis for its proposed relationship to psychogenic pain in children; therefore the utility of further descriptive research on these variables is limited. The variable of coping strategies has a theoretical base and beginning empirical support for its relationship to existing psychogenic pain, but researchers have not studied coping as a mediating factor. Studies of adults have shown that when active coping strategies were ineffective in conditions of uncertainty, muscle tension, cardiac output, and systolic blood pressure increased (Lovallo et al., 1985). Similar studies of coping strategies and concomitant biophysical variables have not yet been done with children. In the future, researchers might prospectively examine young children's appraisal of their own coping strategies with respect to various sources of stress, then observe which children make frequent visits to school health offices for headache, stomachache, limb, or chest pain. A comparison of coping strategies that were predominantly used by symptomatic children versus asymptomatic children might indicate a predictive relationship between coping strategies and symptom development.

BIOPHYSICAL VARIABLES

Genetic Predisposition

Clinicians have noted characteristic fingerprints in individuals with certain gastrointestinal (GI) conditions such as constipation (Staiano, Andreotti, Perrotta, & Striscluglio, 1990). Because patterns of skin ridges (dermatoglyphics) are genetically determined, distinctive dermatoglyphics may indicate a genetic predisposition to GI conditions. Digital whorls and loops in fingerprints are common, while digital arches are rare; all are inherited as autosomal dominant characteristics (Gottlieb & Schuster, 1986) and are permanent by 17 weeks of gestation (Moore, 1988). One investigator found that children who have constipation with and without recurrent abdominal pain had a significantly greater number of digital arches than healthy children, which suggested that some children are genetically predisposed to abdominal pain and/or constipation (Staiano et al., 1990). It is not known if digital arches are predictive of recurrent pain because of some genetic influence, in which case the label "psychogenic" is inappropriate; or if, in the presence of stress, children with digital arches are more likely to manifest psychogenic pain. Embryologically, skin and GI tissues derive from different germ layers: epidermal tissues arise from the ectoderm, and tissues of the GI tract arise from the mesoderm (Moore, 1988); therefore more basic research is needed to clarify the embryological link between dermatoglyphics and GI conditions.

Differential Reactivity to the Stress Response

An untested hypothesis regarding the etiology of RAP is related to the production of endogenous opiates during stress (Gaffney & Gaffney, 1987). Endorphin activity normally increases during homeostatic responses to stress. If endogenous opiates affect the gastrointestinal tract in the same manner as exogenous opiates (i.e., segmental contractions, colon spasm, pain), then children who develop RAP may have an increased susceptibility to the normal release of endogenous opiates during stressful situations. If this hypothesis is true, then RAP is not psychogenic, but organic in origin, according to the definitions provided earlier.

An alternative hypothesis is that RAP is the result of a deficit in autonomic nervous system recovery from stress, although the specific link to the experience of pain is not stipulated. To test the hypothesis, one research team compared responses of children with RAP, hospitalized children, and asymptomatic children to a cold pressor test (Feuerstein et al., 1982). Although there was evidence of autonomic arousal, there were no significant differences between the groups with respect to digital blood volume pulse rates or heart rates based on electrocardiograms, nor was there any evidence of autonomic recovery deficit. It is not likely that laboratory-induced cold pressor tests simulate the typical stressors of childhood, therefore the validity of this line of research is questionable. Another research team measured urinary cortisol, epinephrine, and norepinephrin in school children from specimens taken before and after a major examination, and correlated the results with scores on the investigator-developed Habitual Somatic Discomfort Questionnaire (HSDQ) (Rauste-von Wright & von Wright, 1981). High HSDQ scores correlated with low physiological measures of stress, which suggested that children who somatacize have a *low* physiological reactivity to stress. This study had several measurement weaknesses. The HSDQ had no demonstrated reliability or validity as a measure of somatic symptoms. In addition, the use of one-time biochemical measures is rarely adequate to study complex biophysical processes. The researchers did not take into account the pulsatile release pattern of cortisol, or the circadian rhythm of epinephrine and norepinephrine (Van Cauter & Aschoff, 1989). Finally, the Law of Initial Values must be considered when studying autonomic responses. That is, the magnitude of autonomic response to a stimulus is related to the prestimulus level, and at "extreme initial values, there is a progressive tendency toward 'no response' or 'paradoxic reactions'" (Wilder, 1957, p. 73). Studies are needed in which autonomic and neuroendocrine stress responses are appropriately measured before, during, and after psychogenic pains occur in order to adequately test the reactivity or recovery deficit hypotheses.

Muscle Tension

Theoretically, psychological distress results in muscle tension and headache (Barlow, 1984) or abdominal pain (Rappaport, 1989), but no studies were found in which there was direct measurement of muscle tension before, during, or after a psychogenic pain episode. Based on the assumption that the headaches are due to muscle contraction or tension, several researchers used biofeedback measures and relaxation training protocols to treat children with psychogenic headache. In three studies, subjects were used as their own control, but samples sizes were only 1 (Andrasik et al., 1983); 4 (Engel & Rapoff, 1990); and 31 (Werder & Sargent, 1984). A two-group controlled study had only 11 subjects per group (Larsson & Melin, 1986). Most of the 5- to 12-week training sessions were deemed "successful" at follow-up based on an increased number of pain-free days, and decreased severity and duration of headaches. The regularity with which children continued to use relaxation techniques after initial training sessions relied on self-report, which can be heavily influenced by a social desirability response set. Relaxation protocols have not been reported for symptom management of RAP, limb pain, or chest pain in children.

Although the exact mechanism of transcutaneous electrical stimulation (TENS) is unknown, it has been used with adults to promote relaxation of specific muscles. There is one report of an uncontrolled study in which 29 patients with RAP (ages not stated) placed the TENS unit over the site of the pain, the affected dermatome, or appropriate acupuncture sites. A visual analogue scale was used to measure intensity of pain throughout the study, and the quality of response was based on the percentage of reduction in scores from baseline. At 1–, 3–, and 6–month follow-ups, 72%, 66%, and 52% of the patients, respectively, reported a "good" or "moderately good" response (Sylvester, Kendall, & Lennard-Jones, 1986).

Martin (1983) argued that muscle contraction headache is not a legitimate classification of headaches, citing conflicting research on this topic. For example, in one study of ($n = 47$) 8– to 17–year old children with "problem headaches," obvious muscle contraction versus migraine headache groups did not emerge; each child's attack was very specific and idiosyncratic (Joffe, Bakal, & Kaganov, 1983). Basic empirical work is needed to substantiate the hypothesis that muscle tension is related to psychogenic pain by direct measurement of the tension of related muscle groups before, during, and after a pain epi-sode. Unfortunately, electromyography (EMG) techniques used to measure muscle tension are plagued by multiple sources of error and lack of standards for placement of electrodes and interpretation of findings (Bloch, 1987).

Recurrent Abdominal Pain and Small Bowel Lesions

Much of the clinical diagnostic research on RAP was designed to identify etio-logic factors other than psychogenicity. Ultrasound examinations of the abdo-men showed that in 81% (Shanon, Martin, & Feldman, 1990) to 93.5% (van der Meer, Forget, Arends, Kuijten, & van Engelshoven, 1990) of children with RAP, results were within normal limits. Further, in both studies, none of the few abnormal findings were related to or causative of RAP symptoms.

On the other hand, laboratory tests have been used to test the hypothesis that periumbilical pain experienced by children with RAP may be referred pain from small bowel lesions (van der Meer, Forget, & Heidendal, 1990). Such lesions cause increased permeability of the intestinal wall, which can be indi-rectly measured by higher than normal 24–hour urinary excretion of orally administered chromium labelled ethylene-diaminetetraacetate (Cr-EDTA). In two studies with sample sizes of 87 and 16, children with RAP had a higher percentage of Cr-EDTA excretion than asymptomatic children, and 56% to 66% of children with RAP had clinically significant Cr-EDTA levels (van der Meer et al., 1990, Amery & Forget, 1989). Simultaneous Cr-EDTA measures and biopsies of the lower bowel indicated that the sensitivity of Cr-EDTA is 57%, specificity is 82%, and that lower bowel lesions can be predicted in 89% of the cases (van der Meer, Forget, & Arends, 1990). In one study, children with RAP and high Cr-EDTA excretion were administered drugs to decrease intestinal permeability; the symptoms of all 10 children improved after 1-month admin-istration of oxatomide, a mast-cell stabilizer (Amery & Forget, 1989). Indi-rectly, these studies support an organic basis rather than a psychogenic basis for the abdominal pain. Alternative explanations for increased intestinal per-meability in children with RAP may be that gastrointestinal stress responses weaken the wall of the bowel over time, or that some children are genetically predisposed to increased bowel permeability, which is aggravated by stress re-sponses.

Lactose Malabsorption/Intolerance

Several clinical diagnostic studies were based on the hypothesis that the pain associated with RAP is due to the effects of lactose malabsorption (LM). In six single sample studies of children from the United States (Wald, Chandra, Fisher,

Gartner, & Zitelli, 1982), Canada (Barr, Francoeur, Westwood, & Walsh, 1986; Barr, Watkins, & Perman, 1981), Great Britain (Blumenthal, Kelleher, & Littlewood, 1981), Holland (van der Meer et al., 1990), and Italy (Ceriani et al., 1988), from 12% to 75% of children with RAP (n = 26 to 106) were diagnosed as LM based on lactose breath hydrogen tests. The significance of these results may be misleading in that LM normally occurs in 70% of black Americans, 5% to 20% of whites of Northern European descent (Wald et al., 1982), and in 25% to 50% of the Italian population (Ceriani et al., 1988). In fact, comparative studies showed no difference in the incidence of LM between asymptomatic children and 30 children with RAP (McGrath et al., 1983) or 95 children with chronic diarrhea (Lebenthal, Rossi, Nord, & Branski, 1981).

Related intervention studies were based on the assumption that dietary elimination of lactose-containing products would reduce or eliminate the symptoms, but the results of 6- to 12-week dietary trials are equivocal regarding their effectiveness. Pain episodes decreased significantly from pretrial to posttrial for 18 out of 24 lactose malabsorbers in one study (Ceriani et al., 1988), and there was at least 50% reduction in symptoms for 13 out of 50 subjects in another study (Barr et al., 1986). When malabsorbers were compared to absorbers, however, no significant difference was found in three studies (Blumenthal et al., 1981; Lebenthal et al., 1981; Wald et al., 1982).

Because lactose malabsorption does not occur in many children with RAP, and because symptom reduction may or may not occur with lactose elimination diets, it is likely that RAP and abdominal pain from lactose malabsorption are two separate phenomena. Some clinicians would argue that the lactose breath hydrogen test should be routinely used in the differential diagnosis of abdominal pain in order not to miss the diagnosis, but it would seem that a careful diet history in relationship to the pain episodes would reveal a potential lactose intolerance much less expensively.

Recurrent Abdominal Pain As a Precursor of Organic Syndromes

Some researchers argue that recurrent syndromes in children are migraine equivalents, and are not psychogenic in origin. A retrospective chart review of children with migraines showed that 30% of the children also had RAP (Lanzi et al., 1983) but this small percentage does not adequately support the underlying hypothesis. Studies of visual evoked responses (VER) to red and white light flashes, as indicated on electroencephalogram (EEG) patterns were conducted to test the hypothesis that RAP (sometimes labelled as "abdominal migraine" or "periodic syndrome") in children has a common pathophysiology with childhood migraine headache or with adult's acephalgic migraine. This hypothesis was generally supported by two studies in which, compared to asymptomatic children, both children with RAP and headaches ($n = 28$) (Mortimer & Good, 1990) or periodic syndromes ($n = 8$) (Mortimer, Good, Marsters, & Addy, 1990), and children with migraine had significantly greater than normal VER frequency and amplitude. A controlled study in which 20 children with RAP were treated with antimigraine medication further supported the hypothesis (Symon & Russell, 1986). Seventy percent of the children reported no symptoms, and 30% reported decreases in the frequency of symptoms, whereas 80% of the 20 untreated subjects showed no improvement. An opposing view was offered by Hockaday (1987), who argued that there are no accepted criteria for the diagnosis of "abdominal migraine" and that the diagnosis is too often made by default when organic causes of pain cannot be found. Hockaday also noted that the safety and effectiveness of treatment of RAP with antimigraine medication has an inadequate research base.

RAP has also been considered a precursor to irritable bowel syndrome (IBS) in adults. Adults with IBS have slower than normal gastroduodenal motor activity. When intestinal motility was measured with a semiconductor recording probe, it was found that, despite the small sample size, eight children with RAP had significantly less periodicity, shorter contractions, slower propagation velocity, and greater amplitude of contractions than eight asymptomatic children (Piñeiro-Carrero, Andres, Davis, & Mathias, 1988). It was hypothesized that the decreased intestinal motility and slower movement of intestinal contents causes distention, and that the resultant stimulation of proprioceptors in the intestinal wall causes pain. Adults with IBS have been treated successfully with a high-fiber diet, and two controlled dietary trials for children with RAP showed similar results. A 6–week dietary supplement of fiber cookies resulted in decreased frequency and severity of pain in one-half of the 26 children in the experimental group, but 37% of the placebo group also improved (Feldman, McGrath, Hodgson, Ritter, & Shipman, 1985). The authors indicated that a placebo effect of 25% would be expected. A 7–week liquid fiber dietary trial showed no significant differences in pain episodes between experimental and placebo groups (Christensen, 1986).

In summary, the preceding research has contributed to the list of potential differential diagnoses for pain in children, but has not contributed to an understanding of psychogenic pain. Most intervention research was conducted in the presence of weak evidence of the variable's relationship to psychogenic pain (e.g., muscle tension, small bowel lesions, lactose malabsorption, and RAP as precursors to organic syndromes). Research is needed in which physiological measures are taken *during* pain episodes in order to delineate the actual physiological mechanisms that lead to pain. A comparison of those mechanisms with known pathophysiology of migraine pain would help to refute or support the hypothesis of common pathophysiology.

CONCLUSIONS AND IMPLICATIONS
FOR NURSING RESEARCH

From this body of research, the profile of a child with psychogenic pain emerges: the child is most likely school-age, female, with headache or recurrent abdominal pain, is anxious, and has a low self-esteem. She demonstrates problem behavior at home, but not necessarily at school. Other family members, particularly her mother, have a history of pain and other illnesses. The child has experienced many stressful events in the past year. She will probably continue to have pain or develop other chronic conditions during adulthood. Coleman (1992) proposed a model for psychogenic pain that postulates an etiologic and modulating interaction among 11 variables, many of which were considered in this review. The extant research merely supports the presence of these variables concomitant with symptoms, however, and sheds no light on the interaction among variables nor on the physiologic mechanisms of psychogenic pain. Future research on psychogenic pain in children requires significant changes in all aspects of the research process, including underlying theories, designs, sampling plans, and analyses.

Theory.   Atheoretical descriptive or intervention research delays progress in knowledge development. Variables for study should emanate from theoretical frameworks and relationships among the variables and pain should be logical. Notably absent from any theory was an explanation for the actual experience of *pain*, and exactly *how* pain is related to the variables under study. Although the continued search for alternative etiologies of recurrent pain in children is valuable, such research does not necessarily rule out a "psychogenic" component. Fava and Wise (1987) claimed that the label psychogenic implies linear causality which may be an "a priori error"; rather, researchers should examine "multiple variables that affect a disease process either in its appearance, course, or treatment" (p. 2).

Design.   Qualitative research that describes the experience of pain in children was conspicuously absent; there was no research in which children were asked to reflect on the circumstances surrounding their pain or to describe the pain other than in terms of severity and intensity. The quantitative research was conducted by biologists, sociologists, and psychologists with no apparent collaboration among them. More progress would be made if future research was interdisciplinary, and designed from a biopsychosocial perspective. Researchers with expertise in the reliable and valid measurement of variables should collaborate in order to strengthen the research design. The use of convenience samples should be evaluated. How representative are they? How generalizable are the results from such studies? These teams should avoid the common error of using cursory measures of important variables; such variables should be measured with valid, state-of-the art procedures. Single-subject designs in which subjects act as their own control are useful to observe subtle effects attributable to a treatment that would be missed by group designs (Christophersen, 1982). Finally, there must be more systematic study of the incidence, prevalence, and long-term chronic effects of what has been defined as psychogenic pain in children.

Sample. The lack of consensus on the operational definition of psychogenic pain is one reason for lack of scientific progress. Samples of children with psychogenic pain have been identified on the basis of self-report, parental report, number of pain episodes per time period, or physician diagnosis. To the extent that the operational definitions are different, the sample characteristics may be markedly different. The characteristics of comparison groups were variable, including children who were healthy, or had acute illness, chronic illness, behavior, or psychiatric problems. There is little consensus on the appropriate control or comparison group (Fava & Wise, 1987). Some would argue that because children with psychogenic pain are otherwise physically healthy, the most appropriate comparison group is healthy children who are asymptomatic. It is this author's opinion that the underlying theoretical framework should provide the basis on which comparison groups are selected. Sample sizes should be based on a power analysis or some other logical, verifiable mechanism.

Measurement. Continued examination of single stimulus variables (e.g., stressful life events) or single response variables (e.g., cortisol) will not advance the science. On the other hand, indiscriminant use of multiple measures may be wasteful if they are too highly correlated (Fava & Wise, 1987). More than one method of measuring the same variable is useful if each method has different strengths and limitations. Subjective self-report measures should, when possible, be accompanied by relevant objective measures to control for various response sets. In addition, more careful attention to the reliability and validity of measures, and their sensitivity to change over time is essential. In addition, interobserver reliability checks are essential; one author suggested that 20% of the observations, randomly selected, should be checked (Christophersen, 1982).

Research on psychogenic pain is based on the theory that pain is a physiological response to psychological stress, but no investigators have directly tested the validity of the underlying theory itself. This can only be accomplished by study of the autonomic and endocrine stress responses of children who are experiencing pain. Noninvasive, painless sources of biophysical data are required to decrease the confounding effect of stress related to data collection techniques, particularly with respect to sympathetic and parasympathetic stress responses. Noninvasive techniques that are recommended for use with children include urine and saliva samples as opposed to blood samples (Malamud, 1992; Tunn, Mölmann, Barth, Derendorf, & Dreig, 1992). Finger photoplethysmography is recommended for measurement of cardiovascular responses such as pulse, systolic and diastolic blood pressure (Bloch, 1987). In addition, the r-wave from an electrocardiograph and finger photoplethysmograph can be used as the two points needed to measure pulse transit time.

Although the studies concerned psychogenic pain, pain itself was rarely a variable of interest other than for sample selection. Most researchers did not inquire about the characteristics or quality of the children's pain. In a few studies, investigators included unidimensional pain measures such as visual analogue scales or one-item Likert-type scales for severity and/or intensity. Use of more established, reliable, and valid pain measures appropriate for children would improve the quality of future research (McGrath, 1987).

Investigators who tested an independent variable, or intervention, generally did not describe the intervention in detail. For example, a "relaxation technique" could refer to jaw-slackening, controlled breathing, or systematic total body relaxation techniques. In addition, treatments should not be so laboratory-oriented that they do not generalize to the children's natural environment, for example, biofeedback (Christophersen, 1982). Periodic objective and subjective measures of compliance with treatment are as important as a laboratory's quality control checks. It is strongly recommended that both immediate and long-term effects of a treatment be measured to assure "generality" of treatment effects (Christophersen, 1982).

Analysis. Elementary statistical analyses predominated in the research on children's psychogenic pain. Some investigators failed to acknowledge obvious violations of underlying statistical assumptions. More complex statistical techniques are required to examine the moderating and mediating effects of many variables on psychogenic pain. In addition, theoretical research, using path analysis techniques, are needed. When autonomic response variables are measured, investigators must take into account the Law of Initial Values in data analysis. Prestimulus levels can be controlled through a variety of statistical methods described by Benjamin (1963).

In summary, knowledge about the phenomenon of psychogenic pain in children would be advanced by research that is theoretically based, interdisciplinary, and more rigorous in design, sampling, instrumentation, and data analysis. All aspects of the phenomenon, from incidence to intervention and long-term consequences, require more systematic study to determine the role of psychogenesis in periodic, otherwise unexplained, pain in children.

Nurses, especially school nurses, pediatric clinic nurses, and primary care nurse practitioners, encounter children with RAP on a routine basis. These and other pediatric and primary care clinicians would benefit from an informed and informative literature on this condition. An informed literature would include empirically tested and verified theories on the causes or fundamental mechanisms of RAP, differentiation of types and causative factors if there is more than one type, and development and testing of treatment modalities. Finally, the practice arena would be well served by knowing, from longitudinal studies, what happens to children with RAP as they grow into young adulthood and beyond. Does the condition disappear or does it change into an adult form of disease?

REFERENCES

Adams, J. A., & Weaver, S. J. (1986). Self-esteem and perceived stress in young adolescents with chronic disease. *Journal of Adolescent Health Care, 7,* 173–177.

American Psychiatric Association (1980). *Diagnosis and statistical manual of mental disorders* (3rd edition). Washington, DC: American Psychiatric Press.

Amery, W. K., & Forget, P. P. (1989). The role of the gut in migraine: The oral 51-Cr EDTA test in recurrent abdominal pain. *Cephalalgia, 9,* 227–229.

Andrasik, F., Blanchard, E. B., Edlund, S. R., & Attanasio, V. (1983). EMG biofeedback treatment of a child with muscle contraction headache. *American Journal of Clinical Biofeedback, 6,* 96–102.

Apley, J. (1975). *The child with abdominal pains.* London: Blackwell Scientific Publications.

Apley, J., & Naish, N. (1958). Recurrent abdominal pains: A field survey of 1,000 school children. *Archives of Disease in Childhood, 33,* 165–170.

Astrada, C. A., Licamele, W. L., Walsh, T. L., & Kessler, E. S. (1981). Recurrent abdominal pain in children and associated DSM-III diagnoses. *American Journal of Psychiatry, 138,* 687–688.

Barlow, C. F. (1984). Psychogenic headache. In C. F. Barlow (Ed.), *Headaches and migraine in childhood* (pp. 172–180). Philadelphia: Lippincott.

Barr, R. G., Francoeur, T. E., Westwood, M., & Walsh, S. (1986). Recurrent abdominal pain due to lactose intolerance revisited. *American Journal of Diseases of Childhood, 140,* 302.

Barr, R. G., Watkins, J. B., & Perman, J. A. (1981). Mucosal function and breath hydrogen excretion: Comparative studies in the clinical evaluation of children with nonspecific abdominal complaints. *Pediatrics, 68,* 526–533.

Benjamin, L. S. (1963). Statistical treatment of the Law of Initial Values (LIV) in autonomic research: A review and recommendation. *Psychosomatic Medicine, 25,* 556–566.

Bloch, R. M. (1987). Psychophysiological methods in psychosomatic research. *Advances in Psychosomatic Medicine, 17,* 134–166.

Blumenthal, I., Kelleher, J., & Littlewood, J. M. (1981). Recurrent abdominal pain and lactose intolerance in children. *British Medical Journal, 282,* 2013–2014.

Brunswick, A., Boyle, J., & Tarica, C. (1979). Who sees the doctor? A study of urban black adolescents. *Social Science and Medicine, 13A,* 45–49.

Bury, R. G. (1987). A study of 111 children with recurrent abdominal pain. *Australian Paediatric Journal, 23,* 117–119.

Castleberry, K. (1988). Rules for disease: An interactional model for psychosomatic illness in families. *Issues in Mental Health Nursing, 9,* 363–371.

Ceriani, R., Zuccato, E., Fontana, M., Zuin, G., Ferrari, L., Principi, N., Paccagnini, S., & Mussini, E. (1988). Lactose malabsorption and recurrent abdominal pain in Italian children. *Journal of Pediatric Gastroenterology and Nutrition, 7,* 852–857.

Choquet, M., & Menke, H. (1987). Development of self-perceived risk behaviour and psychosomatic symptoms in adolescents: A longitudinal approach. *Journal of Adolescence, 10,* 291–308.

Christensen, M. F. (1986). Recurrent abdominal pain and dietary fiber. *American Journal of Disease in Childhood, 140,* 738–739.

Christophersen, E. R. (1982). Methodological issues in behavioral pediatrics research. In P. Karoly, J. Steffen, & D. O'Grady (Eds.), *Child health psychology: Concepts and issues* (pp. 104–118). New York: Pergamon Press.

Chu, M. L., & Shinnar, S. (1992). Headaches in children younger than 7 years of age. *Archives of Neurology, 49,* 79–82.

Cohen, J. (1977). *Statistical power analysis for the behavioral sciences.* (Revised ed.). Orlando: Academic Press.

Coleman, W. L. (1984). Recurrent chest pain in children. *Pediatric Clinics of North America, 31,* 1007–1026.

Coleman, W. L. (1992). Recurrent pain and Munchausen syndrome by proxy. In M. D. Levine, W. B. Carey, & A. C. Crocker (Eds.), *Developmental-Behavioral Pediatrics* (pp. 339–349). Philadelphia: Saunders.

Crossley, R. B. (1982). Hospital admissions for abdominal pain in childhood. *Journal of the Royal Society of Medicine, 75,* 772–776.

Davison, I. S., Faull, C., & Nicol, A. R. (1986). Research note: Temperament and behavior in six-year-olds with recurrent abdominal pain: A follow-up. *Journal of Child Psychology and Psychiatry, 27,* 539–544.

Eaton, M. T., Peterson, M. H., & Davis, J. A. (1981). Psychological factors affecting physical conditions. In M. T. Eaton, M. H. Person, & J. A. Davis (Eds.), *Psychiatry* (pp. 181–191). Garden City, NY: Medical Examination Publishing Co.

Engel, J. M., & Rapoff, M. A. (1990). Biofeedback-assisted relaxation training for adult and pediatric headache disorders. *The Occupational Therapy Journal of Research, 10,* 283–299.

Ernst, A. R., Routh, D. K., & Harper, D. C. (1984). Abdominal pain in children and symptoms of somatization disorder. *Journal of Pediatric Psychology, 9,* 77–85.

Faull, C., & Nicol, A. R. (1986). Abdominal pain in six-year-olds: An epidemiological study in a new town. *Journal of Child Psychology and Psychiatry, 47,* 251–260.

Fava, G. A., & Wise, T. N. (1987). Methodological issues in psychosomatic research. *Advances in Psychosomatic Medicine, 17,* 1–2.

Feldman, W., McGrath, P., Hodgson, C., Ritter, H., & Shipman, R. T. (1985). The use of dietary fiber in managing recurrent childhood abdominal pain. *American Journal of Diseases in Children, 139,* 1216–1218.

Feuerstein, M., Barr, R. G., Francoeur, T. E., Houle, M., & Rafman, S. (1982). Potential biobehavioral mechanisms of recurrent abdominal pain in children. *Pain, 13,* 287–298.

Gaffney, A., & Gaffney, P. R. (1987). Recurrent abdominal pain in children and the endogenous opiates: A brief hypothesis. *Pain, 26,* 217–219.

Garber, J., Zeman, J., & Walker, L. S. (1990). Recurrent abdominal pain in children: Psychiatric diagnoses and parental psychopathology. *Journal of the American Academy of Child and Adolescent Psychiatry, 29,* 648–656.

Garmezy, N., & Rutter, M. (1983). *Stress, coping and development in childhood.* New York: McGraw-Hill.

Gascon, G. G. (1984). Chronic and recurrent headaches in children and adolescents. *Pediatric Clinics of North America, 31*, 1028–1051.

Gaylord, N., & Carson, S. (1983). Assessing recurrent abdominal pain in children. *Nurse Practitioner, 8*, 19–?.

Geist, R. (1989). Use of imagery to describe functional abdominal pain as an aid to diagnosis in a pediatric population. *Canadian Journal of Psychiatry, 34*, 506–511.

Gottlieb, S. H., & Schuster, M. M. (1986). Dermatoglyphic (fingerprint) evidence for a congenital syndrome of early onset constipation and abdominal pain. *Gastroenterology, 91*, 428–432.

Greene, J. W., Walker, L. S., Hickson, G., & Thompson, J. (1985). Stressful life events and somatic complaints in adolescents. *Pediatrics, 75*, 19–22.

Haggerty, J. J. (1983). The psychosomatic family: An overview. *Psychosomatics, 24*, 615–618.

Henker, F. O. (1984). Psychosomatic illness: Biochemical and physiologic foundations. *Psychosomatics, 25*, 19–24.

Hockaday, J. M. (1987). Migraine and its equivalents in childhood. *Developmental Medicine and Child Neurology, 29*, 258–270.

Hodges, K., Kline, J. J., Barbero, G., & Flanery, R. (1984). Life events occurring in families of children with recurrent abdominal pain. *Journal of Psychosomatic Research, 28*(3), 185–188.

Hodges, K., Kline, J. J., Barbero, G., & Flanery, R. (1985a). Depressive symptoms in children with recurrent abdominal pain and their families. *Journal of Pediatrics, 107*, 622–626.

Hodges K., Kline J. J., Barbero G., Woodruff C. (1985b). Anxiety in children with recurrent abdominal pain and their parents. *Psychosomatics, 26*, 859–866.

Holmes, T. H., & Masuda, M. (1974). Life change and illness susceptibility. In B. S. Dohrenwend & B. P. Dohrenwend (Eds.), *Stressful life events: Their nature and effects* (pp. 45–72). New York: Wiley.

Hughes, M. C. (1984). Recurrent abdominal pain and childhood depression: Clinical observations of 23 children and their families. *American Journal of Orthopsychiatry, 54*, 146–155.

Jay, G. W., & Tomasi, L. G. (1981). Pediatric headaches: A one year retrospective analysis. *Headache, 21*, 5–9.

Joffe, R., Bakal, D. A., & Kaganov, J. (1983). A self-observation study of headache symptoms in children. *Headache, 23*, 20–25.

Kowal, A., & Pritchard, D. (1990). Psychological characteristics of children who suffer from headache: A research note. *Journal of Child Psychology and Psychiatry, 31*, 637–649.

Lanzi, G., Ballotin, U., Ottolini, A., Rosano Burgio, F., Fazzi, E., & Arisi, D. (1983). Cyclic vomiting and recurrent abdominal pains as migraine or epileptic equivalents. *Cephalgia, 3*, 115–118.

Larsson, B. (1988). The role of psychological, health-behaviour and medical factors in adolescent headache. *Developmental Medicine, 30*, 616–625.

Larsson, B. S. (1991). Somatic complaints and their relationship to depressive symptoms in Swedish adolescents. *Journal of Child Psychology and Psychiatry, 32*, 821–832.

Larsson, B., & Melin, L. (1986). Chronic headaches in adolescents: Treatment in a school setting with relaxation training as compared with information-contact and self-registration. *Pain, 25*, 325–336.

Lazarus, R. S. (1966). *Psychological stress and the coping process.* New York: McGraw-Hill.

Lazarus, R. S. (1991). Stress, coping and illness. In M. Friedman (Ed.), *Personality and diseases* (pp. 97–120). New York: Wiley & Sons.

Lazarus, R. S., & Launier, R. (1978). Stress-related transactions between person and environment. In L. A. Pervin & M. Lewis (Eds.), *Perspectives in Interactional Psychology* (pp. 287–327). New York: Plenum Press.

Lebenthal, E., Rossi, T. M., Nord, K. S., & Branski, D. (1981). Recurrent abdominal pain and lactose absorption in children. *Pediatrics, 67,* 828–832.

Lewis, C. E., & Lewis, M. A. (1989). Educational outcomes and illness behaviors of participants in a child-initiated care system: A 12 year follow-up study. *Pediatrics, 84,* 845–850.

Lewis, C. E., Lewis, M. A., Lorimer, A., & Palmer, B. B. (1977). Child-initiated care: The use of school nursing services by children in an "adult-free" system. *Pediatrics, 60,* 499–507.

Li, B. U. K. (1987). Recurrent abdominal pain in childhood: An approach to common disorders. *Comprehensive Therapy, 13* (10), 46–53.

Lovallo, W. R., Wilson, M. F., Pincomb, G. A., Edwards, G. L., Tompkins, P., & Brackett, D. J. (1985). Activation patterns to aversive stimulation in man. Passive exposure versus effort to control. *Psychophysiology, 22,* 283–291.

Magni, G., Pierri, M., & Donzelli, F. (1987). Recurrent abdominal pain in children: A long term follow-up. *European Journal of Pediatrics, 146,* 72–74.

Malamud, D. (1992). Saliva as a diagnostic fluid. Second now to blood? *British Medical Journal, 305,* 207–208.

Martin, M. J. (1983). Muscle-contraction (tension) headache. *Psychosomatics, 24,* 319–323.

McGrath, P. A. (1987). An assessment of children's pain: A review of behavioral, physiological, and indirect scaling techniques. *Pain, 31,* 147–176.

McGrath, P. J., Goodman, J. T., Firestone, P., Shipman, R., & Peters, S. (1983). Recurrent abdominal pain: A psychogenic disorder? *Archives of Disease in Childhood, 58,* 888–890.

Mechanic, D. (1983). Adolescent health and illness behavior: Review of the literature and a new hypothesis for the study of stress. *Journal of Human Stress, 9* (2), 4–13.

Moore, K. L. (1988). *The developing human* (4th ed.). Philadelphia: Saunders.

Mortimer, M. J., & Good, P. A. (1990). The VER as a diagnostic marker for childhood abdominal migraine. *Headache, 30,* 642–645.

Mortimer, M. J., Good, P. A., Marsters, J. B., & Addy, D. P. (1990). Visual evoked responses in children with migraine: A diagnostic test. *Lancet, 335,* 75–77.

Nader, P. R., & Brink, S. G. (1981). Does visiting the school health room teach appropriate or inappropriate use of health services? Children's use of school health rooms. *American Journal of Public Health, 71,* 416–419.

Naish, J. M., & Apley, J. (1951). "Growing pains": A clinical study of nonarthritic limb pains in children. *Archives of Disease in Childhood, 26,* 134–140.

Page-Goertz, S. (1988). Recurrent abdominal pain in children. *Issues in Comprehensive Pediatric Nursing, 11,* 179–191.

Pantell, R. H., & Goodman, B. W. (1983). Adolescent chest pain: A prospective study. *Journal of Pediatrics, 71,* 881–887.

Passchier, J., & Orlebeke, J. F. (1985). Headaches and stress in school children: An epidemiological study. *Cephalgia, 5,* 167–176.

Peterson, H. (1986). Growing pains. *Pediatric Clinics of North America, 33*, 1365–1372.

Piñeiro-Carrero, V. M., Andres, J. M., Davis, R. H., & Mathias, J. R. (1988). Abnormal gastroduodenal motility in children and adolescents with recurrent functional abdominal pain. *Journal of Pediatrics, 113*, 820–825.

Poole, S. R. (1984). Recurrent abdominal pain in childhood and adolescence. *American Family Physician, 30*, 131–137.

Rappaport, L. (1989). Recurrent abdominal pain: Theories and pragmatics. *Pediatrician, 16*, 78–84.

Rauste-von Wright, M., & von Wright, J. (1981). A longitudinal study of psychosomatic symptoms in healthy 11–18 year old girls and boys. *Journal of Psychosomatic Research, 25*, 525–534.

Raymer, D., Weininger, O., & Hamilton, J. R. (1984). Psychological problems in children with abdominal pain. *Lancet,* Feb. 25, 439–440.

Reynolds, S. L., & Jaffe, D. M. (1990). Children with abdominal pain: Evaluation in the pediatric emergency department. *Pediatric Emergency Care, 6*, 8–12.

Robinson, D. P., Greene, J. W., & Walker, L. S. (1988). Functional somatic complaints in adolescents: Relationship to negative life events, self-concept, and family characteristics. *Journal of Pediatrics, 113*, 588–593.

Robinson, J. O., Alverez, J. H., & Dodge, J. A. (1989). Life events and family history in children with recurrent abdominal pain. *Journal of Psychosomatic Research, 34*, 171–181.

Routh, D. K., & Ernst, A. R. (1984). Somatization disorder in relatives of children and adolescents with functional abdominal pain. *Journal of Pediatric Psychology, 9*, 427–437.

Ryan, N. M. (1986). Recurrent abdominal pain among school-aged children. *American Journal of Maternal Child Nursing, 11*, 102–106.

Ryan, N. M. (1988). The stress-coping process in school-aged children: Gaps in the knowledge needed for health-promotion. *Advances in Nursing Science, 11*(1), 1–12.

Ryan-Wenger, N. M. (1990). Children's psychosomatic responses to stress. In L. E. Arnold (Ed.), *Childhood Stress* (pp. 109–138). New York: Wiley.

Salmon, M. A. (1985). Abdominal migraine in childhood and its place in the evolution of adult (cranial) migraine. *Cephalgia, 5* (Suppl. 3), 182.

Sanders, M. R., Rebgetz, M., Morrison, M., Bor, W., Gordon, A, Dadds, M., & Shepard, R. (1989). Cognitive-behavioral treatment of recurrent nonspecific abdominal pain in children: An analysis of generalization, maintenance and side effects. *Journal of Consulting and Clinical Psychology, 57*, 294–300.

Sawyer, M. G., Davidson, G. P., Goodwin, D., & Crettenden, A. D. (1987). Recurrent abdominal pain in childhood: Relationship to psychological adjustment of children and families: A preliminary study. *Australian Pediatric Journal, 23*, 121–124.

Schechter, N. L. (1984). Recurrent pains in children: An overview and approach. *Pediatric Clinics of North America, 31*, 949–968.

Selbst, S. M. (1985). Chest pain in children. *Pediatrics, 75*, 1068–1070.

Shanon, A., Martin, D. J., & Feldman, W. (1990). Ultrasonographic studies in the management of recurrent abdominal pain. *Pediatrics, 86*, 35–38.

Sharrer, V. W., & Ryan-Wenger, N. M. (1991). Measurements of stress and coping among children with and without recurrent abdominal pain. *Journal of School Health, 61*, 86–91.

Sillanpää, M. (1983a). Changes in the prevalence of migraine and other headaches during the first seven school years. *Headache, 23,* 15–19.

Sillanpää, M. (1983b). Prevalence of headache in prepuberty. *Headache, 23,* 10–14.

Staiano, A., Andreotti, M. R., Perrotta, V., & Striscluglio, P. (1990). Prevalence of digital arches in children with abdominal pain and constipation. *Journal of Pediatrics, 117,* 435–436.

Starfield, B., Gross, E., Wood, M., Pantell, R., Allen, C., et al. (1980). Psychosocial and psychosomatic diagnoses in primary care of children. *Pediatrics, 66,* 159–167.

Starfield, B., Katz, H., Gabriel, A., Livingston, G., Benson, B. A., Harkins, J., Horn, S., & Steinbach, D. (1984). Morbidity in childhood: A longitudinal view. *New England Journal of Medicine, 310,* 824–829.

Stephenson, C. (1983). Visits by elementary school children to the school nurse. *Journal of School Health, 53,* 594–598.

Sylvester, K., Kendall, G. P. N., & Lennard-Jones, J. E. (1986). Treatment of functional abdominal pain by transcutaneous electrical nerve stimulation. *British Medical Journal, 293,* 481–482.

Symon, D. N. K., & Russell, G. (1986). Abdominal migraine: A childhood syndrome defined. *Cephalgia, 6,* 223–228.

Szer, I. S. (1989). Limb pain in healthy children. *Patient Care, 23,* 51–59.

Tunn, S., Mollmann, H., Barth, J., Derendorf, H., & Kreig, M. (1992). Simultaneous measurement of cortisol in serum and saliva after different forms of cortisol administration. *Clinical Chemistry, 8,* 1491–1494.

Van Cauter, E., & Aschoff, J. (1989). Endocrine and other biological rhythms. In L. J. DeGroot (Ed.), *Endocrinology* (2nd ed.) (pp. 2658–2705). Philadelphia: Saunders.

van den Bree, M. B. M., Passchier, J., & Emmen, H. H. (1990). Influence of quality of life and stress coping behaviour on headaches in adolescent male students: An explorative study. *Headache, 30,* 165–168.

van der Meer, S. B., Forget, P. P., & Arends, J. W. (1990). Abnormal small bowel permeability and duodenitis in recurrent abdominal pain. *Archives of Disease in Childhood, 65,* 1311–1314.

van der Meer, S. B., Forget, P. P., Arends, J. W., Kuijten, R. H., & van Engelshoven, J. M. A. (1990). Diagnostic value of ultrasound in children with recurrent abdominal pain. *Pediatric Radiology, 20,* 501–503.

van der Meer, S. B., Forget, P. P., & Heidendal, G. A. K. (1990). Small bowel permeability to 51 Cr-EDTA in children with recurrent abdominal pain. *Acta Paediatrica Scandinavia, 79,* 422–426.

Wald, A., Chandra, R., Fisher, S. T., Gartner, J. C., & Zitelli, B. (1982). Lactose malabsorption in recurrent abdominal pain of childhood. *Journal of Pediatrics, 100,* 65–68.

Walker, L. S., & Greene, J. W. (1989). Children with recurrent abdominal pain and their parents: More somatic complaints, anxiety, and depression than other patient families? *Journal of Pediatric Psychology, 14,* 231–243.

Wasserman, A. L., Whitington, P. F., & Rivara, F. P. (1988). Psychogenic basis for abdominal pain in children and adolescents. *Journal of the American Academy of Child and Adolescent Psychiatry, 27,* 179–184.

Werder, D. S., & Sargent, J. D. (1984). A study of childhood headache using biofeedback as a treatment alternative. *Headache, 24,* 122–126.

Wilder, J. (1957). The law of initial value in neurology and psychiatry: Facts and problems. *Journal of Nervous and Mental Diseases, 125,* 73–86.

Wood, B., Watkins, J. B., Boyle, J. T., Nogueira, J., Zimand, E., & Carroll, L. (1989). The "psychosomatic family" model: An empirical and theoretical analysis. *Family Process*, *28*, 399–417.

Zelasney, B. S. (1990). Understanding recurrent abdominal pain of childhood. *Gastroenterology Nursing*, *13*, 101–104.

Zuckerman, B., Stevenson, J., & Bailey, V. (1987). Stomachaches and headaches in a community sample of preschool children. *Pediatrics*, *79*, 677–682.

Chapter 2

Fatigue During the Childbearing Period

RENÉE A. MILLIGAN
SCHOOL OF NURSING
GEORGETOWN UNIVERSITY

LINDA C. PUGH
SCHOOL OF NURSING
THE JOHNS HOPKINS UNIVERSITY

CONTENTS

Throughout history, fatigue has been recognized as a common accompaniment of pregnancy and the puerperium. Although this is often explained as a result of rapid physiological and psychological changes, few researchers have explored the phenomenon of fatigue during the childbearing experience. The purpose of this chapter is to present an overview of research about fatigue during the childbearing period from the perspective of nursing and related disciplines.

PROCESS FOR REVIEW

A search of nursing and related journals from the past 20 years revealed a number of studies of fatigue in healthy and ill populations but few studies about fatigue during the childbearing period. A thorough review of studies that were focused on fatigue as a concept during childbearing periods (pregnancy, labor, delivery, postpartum) yielded little. Fatigue was seldom an explicit predictor or outcome variable of the research. In research about the childbearing period, however, fatigue was frequently included as an explanatory or intervening construct, sometimes based on subject comments and sometimes based on researcher interpretation. Therefore, studies about childbearing women were evaluated for references to fatigue or similar feelings (weariness, tiredness, lassitude, exhaustion).

This chapter includes general background information about fatigue, and information specific to childbearing fatigue. In order to better understand how childbearing fatigue fits within the overall study of fatigue, insights from ergonomics, medicine, nursing, industry, and psychology provided general information about ways fatigue has been conceptualized and studied. The limited number of studies that were focused on childbearing women's fatigue are reviewed. Many of the references to fatigue in general studies of childbearing women are also included in order to provide contextual insights about how often women experience fatigue within the childbearing experience.

FATIGUE

Fatigue has been defined by researchers in various disciplines including psychology, muscle physiology, ergonomics, and nursing. As a result many conceptualizations of fatigue have emerged but few are directly applicable to nursing care (Piper, 1991). Because little interdisciplinary collaboration exists in fatigue research, a conclusion could be drawn that fatigue has been defined differently for each discipline. All work contributes to a clearer conceptualization of the general construct of fatigue, however (Piper, 1991).

Most definitions of fatigue include all or most of the following dimensions: work decrement, physiologic effects, and feelings of weariness (Bartley & Chute, 1947; Muscio, 1922). In this chapter, the Classification of Nursing Diagnosis (NANDA, 1990) definition of fatigue is used: "An overwhelming sustained sense of exhaustion and decreased capacity for physical and mental work" (p. 73).

Historically, it has been accepted that when fatigued, a person's energy and her use of it are unbalanced as a result of physiological, psychological, or pathophysiological events (Bartley, 1976; Bartley & Chute, 1947; Grandjean,

1970; Hart & Freel, 1982; Muscio, 1921). Fatigue may be an acute or chronic experience characterized by ineffective task performance, self-assured inadequacy, aversion to activity, tiredness or a sense of weariness, body discomfort, and efforts to stop uncomfortable feelings (Sugarman & Berg, 1984; Yoshitake, 1971, 1978). Fatigue is significant when equilibrium cannot be maintained to the point that fatigue adversely affects the person's well-being and interferes with activities of daily living, other activities, and relationships (Aistairs, 1987).

An effort has been made within nursing to synthesize existing research and systematically conceptualize fatigue in nonclinical and specific clinical populations (e.g., Aistairs, 1987; Belza, Henke, Yelin, Epstein, & Gilliss, 1993; Blesch et al., 1991; Piper, 1989, 1991; Piper, Lindsey & Dodd, 1987; Potempa, Lopez, Reid, & Lawson, 1986). Existing nursing frameworks that guide research identify predisposing conditions and causes of fatigue. Rhoten (1982) developed a model of causes of fatigue in postsurgical patients in which fatigue was the end product of the stress response. Piper's (1991) Fatigue Framework in Healthy and Clinical Populations included multiple hypothesized causes of fatigue in specific client populations (e.g., life event patterns, social patterns, activity/rest patterns, disease patterns, and treatment patterns). Potempa et al. (1986) articulated three dimensions of chronic fatigue: physiologic, psychologic, and personality.

In conceptualizing fatigue researchers identified dimensions of fatigue most pertinent to the content area being studied. Most conceptualizations included physiological, psychological, situational, and performance dimensions of fatigue. These four dimensions of fatigue served as the category system for presenting this critical review of studies.

Physiological Dimensions of Fatigue

Fatigue has been defined by physiologists as a decrease in response after prolonged activity (Welford, 1953). The etiology of fatigue is the body's inability to maintain equilibrium when faced with stresses that tax its homeostatic mechanisms (Bartley, 1965, 1967, 1976; Grandjean, 1968, 1969, 1970; Hart & Freel, 1982). Energy imbalance results in feelings of local muscle fatigue, general muscle fatigue, a generalized fatigue state, or a combination. In Poteliakhoff's (1981) physiological model of fatigue, stress causes an increase in plasma cortisol. After a time, exhaustion in hypothalamic cells leads to decreased stimulation of the pituitary-adrenal axis. In Rhoten's (1982) model of fatigue, physiological factors refer to interference with normal body processes, which include malnutrition, inadequate sleep and rest, and medications that drain energy supply. Pathological factors include organic disease processes and pain (Rhoten, 1982).

Various physiologic measures have been used to represent fatigue. These include heart rate, skin and body temperature and heat conductance, sweating, heat loss from the skin, electromyographic (EMG) activity, catecholamine excretion (Kinsman & Weiser, 1976), plasma cortisol levels (Poteliakhoff, 1981), accumulation of lactic acid (Edwards, 1986; Johansson et al., 1987; Sahlin, 1986), muscle ergograms (Schwab, 1953), motor fatigue of arm and leg (Barth, Holding, & Stamford, 1976; Nicklin, Karni, & Wiles, 1987), and occurrence of ketonuria (Courtice & Douglas, 1936).

Psychological Dimensions of Fatigue

Psychologists have identified fatigue as observable within the organism through changes in feelings and behavior (Welford, 1953). Fatigue has been identified as a mood dimension distinct from tension, anxiety, bewilderment, confusion, and depression despite its association with them (Barton, 1978; Curran & Cattell, 1976; Howarth & Schokman-Gates, 1982; Nesselroade, Mitteness & Thompson, 1984; Norcross, Guadagnoli, & Prochaska, 1984). Individuals have been found to be able to discriminate among a variety of mood states, such as anxiety, hostility, depression, and fatigue (Boyle, 1986; Kobashi-Schoot, Hanewald, Van Dam, & Bruning, 1985). Fatigue has also been differentiated from depression in clinical groups. For example, fatigue in multiple sclerosis has been identified as a distinct clinical entity unrelated to depression (Krupp, Alvarez, LaRocca, & Scheinberg, 1988).

From a measurement perspective the constructs can be separated; however, conceptual clarification is sometimes difficult because of fatigue and other psychological conditions, particularly depression and anxiety. Hargreaves (1977) defined the "fatigue syndrome" as a state indistinguishable from an anxiety state with depressive features. The direction of the etiologic relationship between fatigue and depression or anxiety is unclear; depression and anxiety may cause or be caused by fatigue (Potempa et al., 1986). More depression, somatic anxiety, or both are prevalent in fatigued people (Montgomery, 1983). Other emotional factors associated with fatigue include conflicts, frustrations, responsibilities, and worries (Rhoten, 1982). Personality type has also been found to be correlated with fatigue, with some personality types being more vulnerable to fatigue than others (Potempa et al., 1986).

Fatigue has been identified consistently as a symptom of psychiatric disorders such as manic-depressive disorder, or schizophrenia. Fatigue as a symptom of these disorders is not addressed here, as focusing on these disorders in potential research about fatigue during childbearing is beyond the scope of this review.

Situational Dimensions of Fatigue

Situational factors in people's lives have been theorized to be related to fatigue. Examples of these factors are prolonged mental work, monotony, boredom, or environmental factors including illumination, altitude, noise, temperature, and climate (Rhoten, 1982). Feelings of frustration with one's life circumstances have been posited to result in anxiety and psychological and physical over-activity, which in turn lead to depression, inertia, apathy, self-reproach, and fatigue (Davis, 1953). Putt (1975) theorized that the less energy necessary for maintenance of living systems (the less fatiguing the environment), the more energy available for information processing and exchange within the environment.

Performance Dimensions Related to Fatigue

Research about changes in performance generally is based on the assumption that performance accuracy, organization, or speed decrease as fatigue increases (Pritchatt, 1968; Welford, 1953). Fatigue levels are sometimes determined through changes in performance output (Bartley & Chute, 1947; Blitz & Moorst, 1978; Muscio, 1921). Generally, persons stop working when they feel very tired (Kinsman & Weiser, 1976).

Conceptually, definitions of fatigue usually include performance as an indicator. Few nurse investigators have attempted to include performance measures, however. Possibly this is because of the difficulty in quantifying performance. Performance is easily affected by factors other than fatigue, for instance, muscle strength, attitudes, personality, or self-efficacy (Potempa et al., 1986).

Measurement of Fatigue

Kinsman and Weiser (1976) reported three general methods used to measure the subjective symptomology of fatigue. These are: (a) psychophysical approaches, (b) rating scales, and (c) multivariate procedures. In the psychophysical approach, a relationship between the perceived changes in the physical and psychological dimensions of fatigue have been measured in some type of objective units. There are three types of rating scales: (a) nondimensional, (b) unidimensional, and (c) multidimensional. The nondimensional scale assumes fatigue is an all-or-none event, and is considered an imprecise form of measurement. Unidimensional scales such as visual analogs are somewhat stronger; and among available scales, multidimensional measures of fatigue are the most likely to capture the dimensions of this subjective construct.

FATIGUE DURING THE CHILDBEARING PERIOD

Although seldom an a priori variable in research, fatigue or related constructs have been included in the literature about childbearing women. Fatigue often has been identified as an explanatory variable through subjects' reported concerns or researchers' interpretations of subject responses. In pregnancy, fatigue has been related to nausea and vomiting (FitzGerald, 1984), employment (Brown, 1987; Easterbrooks & Goldberg, 1985; Jordan, 1987; Killien & Brown, 1987; Mamelle & Munoz, 1987; Winslow, 1987), or as a symptom during any one of the three trimesters of pregnancy (Fawcett & York, 1986). After childbirth, fatigue has been identified as a concern of new mothers (Drake, Verhulst, & Fawcett, 1988; Fawcett & York, 1986; Gruis, 1977; Guillot, 1964; Harrison & Hicks, 1983; Hazle, 1982; Hiser, 1987; Larsen, 1966; Leifer, 1977; Rubin, 1961, 1975; Sumner & Fritsch, 1977; Tulman & Fawcett, 1988), which is sometimes explained as a symptom of stress or crisis (LeMasters, 1957; Miller & Sollie, 1980; Russell, 1974). During the postpartum period, complaints of fatigue have been related to cesarean delivery (Fawcett, 1981), return to function (Tulman & Fawcett, 1988; Tulman, Fawcett, Groblewski, & Silverman, 1988), needs of multiparous women (Hiser, 1987), breastfeeding (Chapman, Macey, Keegan, Borum, & Bennet, 1985), numbers of children (Hoffman, 1978), infant temperament (Kronstadt, Oberklaid, Ferb, & Swartz, 1979; Panaccione & Wahler, 1986), interference with sexuality (Fischman, Rankin, Soeken, & Lenz, 1986), and as an aspect of postpartum depression or "blues" (Affonso & Domino, 1984; Affonso, Lovett, Paul, & Sheptak, 1990; Beck, Reynolds, & Rutowski, 1992; Carbary, 1982; Pitt, 1975; Robson, 1982).

Since 1989, nurse-investigators have published results of studies focused on fatigue during the childbearing period as an a priori variable. Fatigue has been found to be related to factors during pregnancy (Milligan & Kitzman, 1992; Reeves, Potempa, & Gallo, 1991), during the intrapartum period (Pugh, 1990), and during the postpartum period (Gardner, 1991; Gardner & Campbell, 1991; Milligan, 1989; Milligan, Parks, & Lenz, 1990a). In these studies, fatigue was conceptualized and operationalized in a variety of ways.

Fatigue During Pregnancy

After reviewing a variety of sources, some of which were research-based, Poole (1986) concluded that fatigue is commonly accepted as part of the pregnancy experience. Only two studies were found that were focused on fatigue during pregnancy, however. One strength of each of these studies is that fatigue was clearly defined, and some effort was made to measure it in a manner consistent with its theoretical definition. Reeves, Potempa, and Gallo (1991) proposed that factors such as number and age of children, feeling tired on awakening from sleep, employment, and socioeconomic status were associated with the development of fatigue during pregnancy. In a convenience sample of 20 women, 20–35 years old, few of these factors correlated with fatigue. One exception was that pregnancy fatigue was found to be positively related to nausea and feeling tired upon awakening from sleep. In a study of 74 predominantly African American mothers, Milligan and Kitzman (1992) found depression and anxiety were significantly related to fatigue at 28 and 36 weeks of pregnancy. Anxiety was more strongly related to fatigue than was depression. Each of these studies had small convenience samples, and conclusions were based on simple analytic procedures. Although findings of these investigators suggested ideas for future studies, generalizability was limited.

Although not the focus of research, fatigue surfaced in studies of pregnant women as one among a larger constellation of symptoms. For instance, Fawcett and York (1986) administered a checklist of 20 physical and 3 psychological symptoms to a sample of 70 married couples. In the sample, approximately one-third of the women were in early pregnancy, one-third were in late pregnancy, and one-third were postpartum. Among other symptoms, 91% of the women during early pregnancy and 100% during late pregnancy checked feeling tired.

Mothers also discussed the fatigue that accompanies pregnancy. In a qualitative study (Winslow, 1987) of pregnant women, age 35 to 44, in-depth interviews were conducted with 12 subjects. Older mothers reported that maintaining their full professional schedules during pregnancy was fatiguing. Mothers stated that when they attempted to deal with their fatigue, they realized their lifestyles were changing.

Fatigue has been so commonly accepted during pregnancy that researchers used it to explain other research findings. For instance, DiLorio, van Lier, and Manteuffel (1992) performed a secondary analysis of a sample of 19 white married employed subjects. Their purpose was to ascertain whether a typical pattern of nausea for subjects could be identified. Based on the finding that nausea was most intense in the evening, the authors concluded that fatigue may be an important factor in nausea experiences of working women.

The difficulty in evaluating studies during pregnancy in which fatigue is not the primary focus is that the emphasis of the research was elsewhere, hence little progress on conceptualization or measurement of fatigue emanated from these studies. In these studies, fatigue was measured as a nondimensional construct, and conceptualization was based on the respondent's idiosyncratic perception of fatigue, as in response to the yes/no question, "are you fatigued?"

Fatigue During Labor and Delivery

One study focused on fatigue during the intrapartum period. Pugh (1990) conducted a study of 100 primiparous women interviewed four times during labor and once after delivery. The significant results were that women who were highly anxious, had intravenous pain medication, more childbirth education, less sleep before the onset of labor, and longer labors reported higher fatigue.

This work supported the theory that posits pain medication may influence perception of fatigue (Rhoten, 1982). Women who are medicated during labor often become groggy, more relaxed, and less responsive to stimuli. A significant correlation was also found between the number of hours breathing techniques were used and women's reported fatigue; the longer breathing techniques were used the higher the fatigue. In this study (Rhoten, 1982), multidimensional subjective measurement strategies were used, and unlike any other reported study, a physical indicator to measure fatigue was used (bulb dynamometer). The convenience sample of predominantly white, upper-middle class women makes it difficult to generalize; however, the findings suggest hypotheses for future research.

One other study was reported that provided information about intrapartum fatigue. Lederman, Lederman, Work, and McCann (1985) studied anxiety and stress during labor, using plasma catecholamine levels to operationalize anxiety. In their study of 73 multigravid women, the conclusion was drawn that anxiety and epinephrine levels were positively related to length of labor. This finding may have implications for knowledge generation about fatigue. A fatigue-anxiety relationship (Montgomery, 1983; Rhoten, 1982) has been posited. Catecholamine levels have been used as physiological indicators of fatigue (Poteliakhoff, 1981).

Postpartum Fatigue

The most frequent complaint of new mothers has been posited to be fatigue (Carbary, 1982). Carbary's statement has been validated by the frequency with which fatigue is mentioned by mothers in studies of postpartum. Fawcett and York (1986) found that 65% of mothers in the postpartum group reported feeling tired. Fawcett (1981), from a retrospective exploratory survey of the needs of 24 couples after cesarean deliveries, found that mothers who had cesarean births after labor identified extreme fatigue as a major problem. Chapman et al. (1985), using a convenience sample of 50 healthy breastfeeding mothers, found that fatigue was a major complaint of subjects through 4 months postpartum.

Other studies that were focused on other aspects of the postpartum period included fatigue as a correlate to characteristics of the mothers. For instance, mothers who had only one child gave more fatigue responses than mothers who had three or more children (Hoffman, 1978). In contrast, Larsen (1966) and Gruis (1977) found that fatigue was of major concern for multiparas, 19 of 23 citing it as a foremost concern.

Reports of tiredness or fatigue surfaced in studies about return to normal functioning after childbirth. After studying 70 women, Tulman and Fawcett (1988) suggested that resuming activities and assuming responsibility for the care of infants (even though they had not returned to prepregnancy functioning) may account for anecdotal reports of prolonged fatigue following child-birth. Tulman and colleagues (1990) studied 97 women over a 6-month period. They reported that lower physical energy was related to less optimal functional status at 3 weeks, 6 weeks, and at 6 months postpartum.

The difficulty in evaluating studies of postpartum women in which fatigue was not the primary focus of the study is that conceptualization and measurement of fatigue is inconsistent. As in studies of pregnancy, fatigue generally was measured as a nondimensional construct, and conceptualized based on the respondent's own interpretation of fatigue. Although, as discussed (Kinsman & Weiser, 1976), the nondimensional single point measures are considered to be the least precise form of measurement, these measures are typically used with postpartum fatigue. Mothers identified postpartum fatigue as important through card-sorting important concerns, one of which was "feeling tired" (Hiser, 1987). Postpartum fatigue was identified through checklists of postpartum concerns, one option of which was fatigue or tiredness (Fawcett & York, 1986; Gruis, 1977; Harrison & Hicks, 1983). The importance of postpartum fatigue was emphasized through relating fatigue to other postpartum issues, as in how much do "my feelings of fatigue interfere with our making love?" (Fischman et al., 1986). Postpartum fatigue was counted as the number of times that mothers mentioned fatigue or tiredness in qualitative descriptions of their postpartum experience (Chapman et al., 1985; Errante, 1985; Fawcett, 1981; Merilo, 1988). Postpartum fatigue was assumed from nurses' prior experience with many postpartum women (Rubin, 1961, 1975; Sumner & Fritsch, 1977). Conceptional and measurement issues are critical to further study of postpartum fatigue, and to some extent have been addressed in the two studies that were focused on postpartum fatigue.

Other weaknesses of studies of postpartum not specifically focused on fatigue revolve around research methods. Many have small samples that are inadequate for complex analysis. Descriptive analysis, the predominant approach used in these studies, does not permit explanation or prediction. Further, external validity may be threatened because of the reliance in most of these studies on homogeneous convenience samples. These generalized weaknesses also were reflected in the studies focusing on postpartum fatigue.

Milligan and colleagues (1990a) studied 259 normal new mothers at the immediate postpartum period, at 6 weeks postpartum, and at 3 months postpartum. Quota sampling was used to provide a sample with a mix of middle- and low-socioeconomic status women. Fatigue was measured using a multidimensional instrument (a modified Fatigue Symptom Checklist based on Yoshitake, 1978), which was consistent with fatigue conceptualization as a negative, multidimensional, subjective experience. Depression was statistically controlled for in the multiple regression analysis. The analytic model was designed to address a variety of dimensions of new mothers' lives, such as age, parity, socioeconomic status, type of feeding, length of labor, and infant diffi-culty. A significant correlation between fatigue during the postpartum hospi-talization and type of delivery was reported: postcesarean section mothers had higher fatigue. At 6 weeks postpartum, higher fatigue was related to type of infant feeding, with breastfeeding mothers being more fatigued. Socioeconomic status at 3 months postpartum was found to be related to postpartum fatigue (controlling for depression), with higher fatigue related to middle, rather than low socioeconomic status. Infant difficulty was also a significant predictor of fatigue (controlling for depression) at 6 weeks postpartum and 3 months post-partum. In this study, an effort was made to follow mothers longitudinally, and to clarify fatigue as a construct separate from depression. The correlations re-ported, although significant, accounted for a small part of the variance in fa-tigue, after the variance for depression was statistically controlled. In a follow-up paper, Milligan, Parks, and Lenz (1990b) posited that although postpartum fatigue and depression did have some overlap, these constructs could be clearly differentiated through studying patterns of change over time and comparing relationships with other variables.

Gardner (1991) also conducted a longitudinal study that was focused on postpartum fatigue, using a convenience sample of predominantly white, mar-ried mothers of normal infants. There was some difficulty with subject attri-tion. At the immediate postpartum period, there were 68 subjects, at 2 weeks postpartum there were 47 subjects, and at 6 weeks, only 35 subjects remained in the study. Fatigue was measured unidimensionally and multidimensionally using the unidimensional visual analog Rhoten scale (1982), and a 3-item fatigue subscale taken from the Beck Depression Inventory (BDI) (Beck, Ward, Mendelson, Mock, & Erbaugh, 1961). In this research, an effort was made to separate the construct of postpartum fatigue from postpartum depression. Fatigue levels as measured by the three item BDI subscale changed significantly among 2 days, 2 weeks, and 6 weeks postpartum, whereas the BDI depression score on the items not in the subscale did not change. The Rhoten fatigue scale scores also did not change significantly across the time periods. Clear separation of fatigue and depression as constructs is difficult based on these findings because the two types of fatigue measures did not reflect similar patterns over the three time periods. The approach was creative, however, and perhaps with some modifica-tion, warrants further research with larger samples. In another report from this study, Gardner and Campbell (1991) reported on the sample of 68 women at 2 days postpartum who completed a visual analog scale rating their fatigue. Based on insights gained from this analysis, the researchers concluded that women with higher fatigue were younger, married, with low income, had two to three other children, less education, less household help, and childcare problems. Sample size was small, and conveniently obtained, which limits generalizability. Many of the relationships identified suggest direction for future study, however.

In another study of the postpartum period Robson (1982) interviewed primiparous women ($n = 119$) once each trimester and four times after birth. In the qualitative analysis of mothers' responses, mothers mentioned fatigue-like symptoms in two ways: as a symptom of postpartum depression and as a symptom separate from postpartum depression. As emphasized in these studies, clarifying the relationship between postpartum fatigue and depression is critical to understanding postpartum fatigue.

SUMMARY AND ANALYSIS OF METHODOLOGIES USED

Fatigue in women during the childbearing period is a pervasive phenomenon. Although strategies for measurement of fatigue were found to be inconsistent, the construct of fatigue was mentioned in many descriptive studies of childbearing. Recent research was found in which childbearing fatigue was the major focus. This descriptive research portrayed fatigue as a robust construct in the lives of women during the childbearing period, one that changed over time, and was related to a variety of other variables in mothers' lives. Much of the research that was focused on fatigue during childbearing provided descriptive, substantive information about a phenomenon that was previously widely accepted but never clarified.

Limitations in studies focused on childbearing fatigue were consistent with beginning research in any area of study. Conceptualization and measurement were inconsistent; however, these problems are pervasive in general study of fatigue. As research designs were limited to descriptive-correlational, no causal relationships could be determined. Direction of predictive relationships among fatigue and other variables, although assumed, were not explicated. For instance, does type of infant feeding predict fatigue levels, or do fatigued mothers choose not to breastfeed? Sample sizes in studies of childbearing fatigue were relatively small. Among studies, diversity in the samples (white, black, high risk, suburban, inner city) was noted, which supports the pervasiveness of the phenomenon. Nonrandom sampling techniques limit the generalizability of findings to the population of childbearing women. According to standards of subjective fatigue measurement (Kinsman & Weiser, 1976), few studies used the most highly recommended multidimensional measures. Attention to psychometric properties of instruments was reported by Milligan et al. (1990b) and Pugh (1993), as was attention to construct validity (Gardner, 1991).

RECOMMENDATIONS FOR RESEARCH

Fatigue during the childbearing period continues to be an understudied topic. Review of the available literature revealed that women's fatigue is pervasive during the childbearing period, both by the number of times that it surfaced in general work about childbearing and based on findings of the few studies that focused on childbearing fatigue.

Need for further research about childbearing fatigue became apparent as past study was evaluated. Childbearing fatigue research to date has generally not attempted to distinguish between acute and chronic fatigue, a categorization found useful in studies of cancer-related fatigue (Piper, 1991). Patterns of how fatigue develops and dissipates during the childbearing period have not been studied. Also, fatigue researchers have not identified the cumulative or interactive effect of different factors on fatigue. It is not known whether fatigue is childbearing-phase specific. Little is known about whether women who experience fatigue during pregnancy are more vulnerable to fatigue in the postpartum period and whether a composite of factors intensifies the vulnerability to fatigue. Research has also not identified the processes that may act as mediators of the effect of those factors on fatigue.

Although there is a need to clarify the construct of childbearing fatigue descriptively, a current gap in the research is also seen in the absence of experimental studies that delineate strategies for preventing or ameliorating fatigue. Because fatigue is pervasive during all phases of the childbearing period, nurse investigators may uncover ways to intervene that dissipate the intensity or frequency of this experience.

The studies needed to fill the gaps in the research about childbearing fatigue would require extensive resources. A longitudinal study that tracks fatigue throughout each phase of childbearing is warranted. In this study, a large diverse sample and fatigue measurement using multidimensional instruments could validate anecdotal knowledge. Currently anecdotal knowledge is the basis of childbearing nursing care activities. Exploratory efforts in conceptualization and measurement of performance dimensions of fatigue could provide background for expansion of what is known about fatigue measurement. After this measurement and descriptive work is complete, well-grounded experimental nursing intervention studies to prevent or ameliorate fatigue could follow. Valid intervention studies would provide the basis for improving nursing practice in the care of childbearing women.

REFERENCES

Affonso, D. D., & Domino, G. (1984). Postpartum depression: A review. *Birth, 11*, 231–235.

Affonso, D. D., Lovett, S., Paul, S. & Sheptak, S. (1990). A standardized interview that differentiates pregnancy and postpartum symptoms from perinatal clinical depression. *Birth, 17*, 121–130.

Aistairs, J. (1987). Fatigue in the cancer patient: a conceptual approach to a clinical problem. *Oncology Nursing Forum, 14*(6), 25–30.

Barth, J. L., Holding, D. H., & Stamford, B. A. (1976). Risk versus effort in the assessment of motor fatigue. *Journal of Motor Behavior, 3*, 189–194.

Bartley, S. H. (1965). *Fatigue: Mechanisms and management.* Springfield, IL: Charles C Thomas.

Bartley, S. H. (1967). *The human organism as a person.* Philadelphia: Chilton.

Bartley, S. H. (1976). What do we call fatigue? In E. Simonson & P. C. Weiser, *Psychological aspects and physiological correlates of work and fatigue* (pp. 409–414). Springfield, IL: Charles C Thomas.

Bartley, S., & Chute, E. (1947). *Fatigue and impairment in men.* New York: McGraw-Hill.

Barton, K. (1978). Psychological mood states in children related to performance on a perceptual motor task. *Multivariate Experimental Clinical Research, 3*, 219–231.

Beck, C. T., Reynolds, M. A., & Rutowski, P. (1992). Maternity blues and postpartum depression. *JOGNN: Journal of Obstetric, Gynecologic, and Neonatal Nursing, 21*, 287–293.

Beck, A. T., Ward, C., Mendelson, M., Mock, J., & Erbaugh, J. (1961). An inventory for measuring depression. *Achives of General Psychiatry, 4*, 561–576.

Belza, B. L., Henke, C. J., Yelin, E. H., Epstein, W. V., & Gilliss, C. L. (1993). Correlates of fatigue in older adults with rheumatoid arthritis. *Nursing Research, 42*, 93–99.

Blesch, K. S., Paice, J. A., Wickham, R., Harte, N., Schnoor, D. K., Purl, S., Rehwalt, M., Kopp, P. L., Manson, S., Coveny, S. B., McHale, M., & Cahill, M. (1991). Correlates of fatigue in people with breast or lung cancer. *Oncology Nursing Forum, 18*, 81–87.

Blitz, P. S., & Moorst, A. V. (1978). Physical fatigue and the perception of differences in load: a signal detection approach. *Perceptual and Motor Skills, 46*, 779–790.

Boyle, G. J. (1986). Analysis of topological factors across the eight-state questionnaire and the differential emotions scale. *Psychological-Reports, 59*, 503–510.

Brown, M. A. (1987). Employment during pregnancy: Influences on women's health and social support. *Health Care for Women International, 8*, 151–167.

Carbary, L. J. (1982). Postpartum depression. *Journal of Nursing Care, 15*(7), 11–13.

Chapman, J. J., Macey, M. J., Keegan, M., Borum, P., & Bennett, S. (1985). Concerns of breast-feeding mothers from birth to 4 months. *Nursing Research, 34*, 374–377.

Courtice, F. C., & Douglas, C. G. (1936). The effects of prolonged muscular exercise on the metabolism. *Procedures of the Royal Society, 119*, 381–439.

Curran, J. R., & Cattell, R. B. (1976). *Handbook for the eight state questionnaire.* Champaign, IL: Institute for Personality and Ability Testing.

Davis, R. D. (1953). Satiation and frustration as determinants of fatigue. In W. F. Floyd & A. T. Welford (Eds.), *Fatigue* (pp. 152–154). London: H. K. Lewis.

DiLorio, C. van Lier, D., & Manteuffel, B. (1992). Patterns of nausea during the first trimester of pregnancy. *Clinical Nursing Research, 1*, 127–140.

Drake, M. L., Verhulst, D., & Fawcett, J. (1988). Physical and psychological symptoms experienced by Canadian women and their husbands during pregnancy and the postpartum. *Journal of Advanced Nursing, 13*, 436–40.

Easterbrooks, M. A., & Goldberg, W. A. (1985). Effects of early maternal employment on toddlers, mothers, and fathers. *Developmental Psychology, 21*, 774–783.

Edwards, R. H. (1986). Interaction of chemical with electromechanical factors in human skeletal muscle fatigue. *Acta Physiologica Scandinavica, 556,* 149–155.

Errante, J. (1985, January). Sleep deprivation or postpartum blues? *Topics in Clinical Nursing, 6*(4), 9–18.

Fawcett, J. (1981). Needs of cesarean birth parents. *JOGNN: Journal of Obstetrics, Gynecologic, and Neonatal Nursing, 10,* 372–376.

Fawcett, J., & York, R. (1986). Spouses' physical and psychological symptoms during pregnancy and the postpartum. *Nursing Research, 35,* 144–146.

Fischman, S. H., Rankin, E. A., Soeken, K. L., & Lenz, E. R. (1986). Changes in sexual relationships in postpartum couples. *JOGNN: Journal of Obstetrics, Gynecologic, and Neonatal Nursing, 15,* 58–63.

FitzGerald, C. M. (1984). Nausea and vomiting in pregnancy. *British Journal of Medical Psychology, 57,* 159–165.

Gardner, D. (1991). Fatigue in postpartum women. *Applied Nursing Research, 4,* 57–62.

Gardner, D. L., & Campbell, B. (1991). Assessing postpartum fatigue, *MCN: The American Journal of Maternal Child Nursing, 16,* 264–266.

Grandjean, E. P. (1968). Fatigue: Its physiological and psychological significance. *Ergonomics, 11,* 427–436.

Grandjean, E. (1969). *Fitting the task to the man—an ergonomic approach.* London: Taylor and Francis.

Grandjean, E. P. (1970). Fatigue. *American Industrial Hygiene Association Journal, 31,* 401–411.

Gruis, M. (1977). Beyond maternity: Postpartum concerns of mothers. *MCN: The American Journal of Maternal Child Nursing, 2,* 182–188.

Guillot, E. (1964). Patterns of help for postpartum mothers. *Children, 11,* 147–151.

Hargreaves, M. (1977). The fatigue syndrome. *Practitioner, 218,* 841–843.

Harrison, M. J., & Hicks, S. A. (1983). Postpartum concerns of mothers and their sources of help. *Canadian Journal of Public Health, 74,* 325–327.

Hart, L. K., & Freel, M. I. (1982). Fatigue. In C. Norris, (Ed.), *Concept clarification in nursing* (pp. 251–262). Rockville: Aspen.

Hazle, N. R. (1982). Postpartum blues: Assessment and intervention. *Journal of Nurse-Midwifery, 27*(6), 21–25.

Hiser, P. L. (1987). Concerns of multiparas during the second postpartum week. *JOGNN: Journal of Gynecologic and Neonatal Nursing, 16,* 195–203.

Hoffman, L. W. (1978). Effects of the first child on the woman's role. In W. B. Miller & L. I. Newman (Eds.), *The first child and family formation* (pp. 340–367). Chapel Hill: Carolina Population Council.

Howarth, E., & Schokman-Gates, K. L. (1982). Manipulated changes across ten mood dimensions. *Personality and Individual Differences, 3,* 211–214.

Johansson, C., Gerdle, B., Lorentzon, R., Rasmuson, S., Reiz, S., & Fugl-Meyer, A. R. (1987). Fatigue and endurance of lower extremity muscles in relation to running velocity at OBLA in male orienteers. *Acta Physiologica Scandinavica, 131,* 203–209.

Jordan, P. (1987). Differences in network structure, social support, and parental adaptation associated with maternal employment status. *Health Care for Women International, 8*(2–3), 133–150.

Killien, M., & Brown, M. A. (1987). Work and family roles of women: Sources of stress and coping strategies. *Health Care for Women International, 8,* 169–184.

Kinsman, R. A., & Weiser, P. C. (1976). Subjective symptomatology during work and fatigue. In E. Simonson & P. C. Weiser (Eds.), *Psychological aspects and physi-*

ological correlates of work and fatigue (pp. 336–405). Springfield, IL: Charles C Thomas.

Kobashi-Schoot, J., Hanewald, G., Van Dam, F., & Bruning, P. (1985). Assessment of malaise in cancer patients treated with radiotherapy. *Cancer Nursing, 8*, 306–313.

Kronstadt, D., Oberklaid, F., Ferb, T. E., & Swartz, J. P. (1979). Infant behavior and maternal adaptations in the first six months of life. *American Journal of Orthopsychiatry, 49*, 454–464.

Krupp, L. B., Alvarez, L. A., LaRocca, N. G., & Scheinberg, L. C. (1988). Fatigue in multiple sclerosis. *Archives of Neurology, 45*, 435–437.

Larsen, V. (1966). Stresses of the childbearing year. *American Journal of Public Health, 56*, 32–36.

Lederman, R. P., Lederman, E., Work, B., & McCann, D. S. (1985). Anxiety and epinephrine in multiparous women in labor: Relationship to duration of labor and fetal heart rate pattern. *American Journal of Obstetrics and Gynecology, 153*, 870–877.

Leifer, M. (1977). Psychological changes accompanying pregnancy and motherhood. *Genetic Psychology Monographs, 95*, 55–96.

LeMasters, E. (1957). Parenthood as a crisis. *Marriage and Family Living, 19*, 352–355.

Mamelle, N., & Munoz, F. (1987). Occupational working conditions and preterm birth: A reliable scoring system. *American Journal of Epidemiology, 126*, 150–152.

Merilo, K. F. (1988). Is it better the second time around? *MCN: The American Journal of Maternal Child Nursing, 13*, 200–204.

Miller, B., & Sollie, D. (1980). Normal stresses during the transition to parenthood. *Family Relations, 29*, 459–465.

Milligan, R. (1989). Maternal fatigue during the first three months of the postpartum period. *Dissertation Abstracts International, 50*, 07–B.

Milligan, R., & Kitzman, H. (1992). Fatigue during pregnancy. Paper presentation at *Nursing Research Across the Life Span: Methods, Issues and Interventions.* Johns Hopkins University and University of Maryland at Baltimore. Baltimore, MD, March 2.

Milligan, R., Parks, P., & Lenz, E. (1990a). An analysis of postpartum fatigue over the first three months of the postpartum period. In J. Wang, P. Simoni, & C. Nath (Eds.). *Vision of excellence: The decade of the nineties* (pp. 245–251). Charleston, WV: West Virginia Nurses' Association Research Conference Group.

Milligan, R., Parks, P., & Lenz, E. (1990b). Measuring postpartum fatigue. Paper presentation at NAACOG National Research Conference: *Making a Difference in Women's and Infants' Health.* Denver, Colorado, July 20–21.

Montgomery, G. K. (1983). Uncommon tiredness among college undergraduates. *Journal of Counseling and Clinical Psychology, 51*, 517–525.

Muscio, B. (1921). Is a fatigue test possible? *British Journal of Psychology, 12*, 31–46.

Nesselroade, J. R., Mitteness, L. S., & Thompson, L. K. (1984). Older adulthood. *Research on Aging, 6*, 3–23.

Nicklin, J., Karni, Y., & Wiles, C. (1987). Shoulder abduction fatiguability. *Journal of Neurology, Neurosurgery, and Psychiatry, 50*, 423–427.

Norcross, J. C., Guadagnoli, E., & Prochaska, J. D. (1984). Factor structure of the profile of mood states (POMS): Two partial replications. *Journal of Clinical Psychology, 40*, 1270–1277.

North American Nursing Diagnosis Association (1990). Taxonomy I revisited - 1990 with official Nursing Diagnoses. St. Louis: Author.

Panaccione, V. F., & Wahler, R. G. (1986). Child behavior, maternal depression, and social coercion as factors in the quality of child care. *Journal of Abnormal Child Psychology, 14*, 263–278.

Piper, B. (1989). Current bases for practice. In S. Funk, E. Tornquist, M. Champagne, L. Copp, & R. Wiese (Eds.). *Key aspects of comfort.* New York: Springer Publishing Co.

Piper, B. (1991). Alterations in energy: The sensation of fatigue. In S. Baird, R. McCorkle, & M. Grant (Eds.), *Cancer nursing: A comprehensive textbook,* (pp. 894–908). Philadelphia: W. B. Saunders Company.

Piper, B., Lindsey, A., & Dodd, M. (1987). Fatigue mechanisms in cancer patients: Developing nursing theory. *Oncology Nursing Forum, 14*(6), 17–23.

Pitt, B. (1975, April). The aftermath of childbirth. *Procedures of the Royal Society of Medicine, 68*, 223–224.

Poole, C. (1986). Fatigue during the first trimester of pregnancy. *JOGNN: Journal of Obstetric, Gynecologic and Neonatal Nurses, 15*, 375–379.

Poteliakhoff, A. (1981). Adrenocortical activity and some clinical findings in acute and chronic fatigue. *Journal of Psychosomatic Research, 25*, 91–95.

Potempa, K., Lopez, M., Reid, C., & Lawson, L. (1986). Chronic fatigue. *Image, 18*, 165–169.

Pritchatt, D. (1968). An investigation into some of the underlying associative verbal processes of the Stroop colour effect. *Quarterly Journal of Experimental Psychology, 18*, 351–359.

Pugh, L. C. (1990). Psychophysiological correlates of fatigue during childbirth. *Dissertation Abstracts International, 51*, 01–B.

Putt, A. (1975). Effects of noise on fatigue in healthy middle-aged adults. *Communicating Nursing Research, 8*, 24–40.

Reeves, N., Potempa, K., & Gallo, A. (1991). Fatigue in early pregnancy. *Journal of Nurse-Midwifery, 36*, 303–309.

Rhoten, D. (1982). Fatigue and the postsurgical patient. In C. Norris (Ed.), *Concept clarification in nursing,* (pp. 277–300). Aspen: Rockville, MD.

Robson, K. M. (1982)). An anxious time. *Nursing Mirror, 154*(23), 14–17.

Rubin, R. (1961). Basic maternal behavior. *Nursing Outlook, 9*, 683–686.

Rubin, R. (1975). Maternity nursing stops too soon. *American Journal of Nursing, 75*, 1680–1684.

Russell, C. (1974). Transition to parenthood: Problems and gratifications. *Journal of Marriage and the Family, 36*, 294–302.

Sahlin, K. (1986). Muscle fatigue and lactic acid accumulation. *Acta Physiologica Scandanavica, 556*, 83–91.

Schwab (1953). Motivation in Measurements of Fatigue. In W. F. Floyd & A. T. Welford (Eds.), *Fatigue* (pp. 143–148). London: H. K. Lewis.

Sugarman, J. R., & Berg, A. O. (1984). Evaluation of fatigue in a family practice. *The Journal of Family Practice, 19*, 643–647.

Sumner, G., & Fritsch, J. (1977). Postnatal parental concerns: the first six months of life. *JOGNN: Journal of Obstetrics, Gynecologic, and Neonatal Nursing, 6*, 27–32.

Tulman, L., & Fawcett, J. (1988). Return of functional ability after childbirth. *Nursing Research, 37*, 77–81.

Tulman, L., Fawcett, J., Groblewski, L., & Silverman, L. (1990). Changes in functional status after childbirth. *Nursing Research, 39*, 70–75.

Welford, A. T. (1953). The psychologist's problem in measuring fatigue. In W. F. Floyd, & A. T. Welford, (Eds.), *Fatigue* (pp. 183–191). London: H. K. Lewis.

Winslow, W. (1987). First pregnancy after 35: What is the experience? *MCN: The American Journal of Maternal Child Nursing, 12,* 92–96.

Yoshitake, H. (1971). Relations between the symptoms and the feeling of fatigue. *Ergonomics, 14,* 175–186.

Yoshitake, H. (1978). Three characteristic patterns of subjective fatigue symptoms. *Ergonomics, 21,* 231–233.

Chapter 3

Elder Mistreatment

TERRY T. FULMER
SCHOOL OF NURSING
COLUMBIA UNIVERSITY

CONTENTS

It is estimated that between 700,000 and 1.2 million elderly individuals in this country are victims of elder mistreatment annually (Pillemer & Finkelhor, 1989). Elder mistreatment, the outcome of abuse, neglect, exploitation, and abandonment, is a prevalent, serious, and morbid syndrome that is poorly recognized and underresearched.

This chapter provides a critical analysis of the elder mistreatment literature since its recognition in the late 1970s. This includes a discussion of the conceptual/ theoretical models of causation, research related to assessment and detection of elder mistreatment, and research-based practice protocols for treatment.

Sources for the relevant studies were identified through a comprehensive review of citations using the Columbia University Health Sciences Library database services. Included were MEDLINE from 1975 through 1992 Cumulative Index of Nursing and Allied Health Literature (CINAHL) 1983 to 1992, database of child abuse and neglect in family violence 1964 to 1992 (from the National Center for the Prevention of Child Abuse), Psych Info 1967 to 1992, Sociological Abstracts 1963 to 1992, and Health Planning and Administration abstracts 1975 to 1992. Key words included elder, abuse, mistreatment, and violence. Checks were conducted to remove duplications from the databases. A total of 660 citations were printed with a resultant review of the abstracts and relevant papers. In addition to abstracting services, the author used the ancestry approach given long term involvement in the field. Data-based articles, written in English, comprised the literature for this review.

An attempt has been made to integrate research in a way that summarizes and critiques the state of knowledge related to elder mistreatment, highlights the major unresolved issues, and makes comments related to future research. For the purpose of this chapter, elder mistreatment will be used as the overarching defining concept, with abuse, neglect, exploitation, and abandonment as operational subsets of the outcome of mistreatment.

OVERVIEW OF THE ELDER MISTREATMENT RESEARCH

Elder mistreatment has evolved as the distinct subsection of the family violence literature over the past 15 years and the literature to date has come from two sources: the sociological/psychological literature and the clinical/disciplinary view. In the former group, as is expected, sociologic and psychologic frameworks have been applied in order to address the problem, whereas in the latter, clinical observation and mandatory reporting laws have largely influenced the nature and approach to research. With specific regard to professional nursing, research has been focused on theoretical formulations of the cause of elder mistreatment, definitional/conceptual frameworks, and clinical assessment and detection efforts including instrument development, instrumentation, and psychometric activity.

Quinn and Tomita (1986) have described research in elder mistreatment in terms of "first- and second-wave" research. This is a commonly held view: the early wave of elder mistreatment research that began in the late 1970s was the ground-breaking work that brought the phenomenon to public attention. During those early years, research was centered around identifying victims and documenting the problem. This first wave of research is believed to have emerged for two reasons: (a) response to new mandatory elder abuse reporting laws; and (b) a genuine recognition of elders as victims. Individuals responsible for early research include Block and Sinnott (1979), Douglass and Hickey (1981), Lau and Kosberg (1978), and O'Malley, Segars, Perez, Mitchell, and Knuepel (1978). From these four seminal studies, Callahan (1986) was moved to say:

> elder abuse is a problem that cannot be defined, cannot be measured accurately, and cannot be isolated for treatment purposes from other clinical and social interventions, and is now, apparently, too confusing and expensive to generate political support. (p. 2)

Since that time, second-wave research has emerged that is teaching us about the phenomenon. Second-wave research is meant to refer to the studies that were designed with theoretical frameworks, rigorous design, and appropriate methods. These include random sample surveys, instrumentation work, and case-control studies.

Elder mistreatment exists, it is serious, and it warrants empirical studies to determine the answers to the questions posed by Callahan (1988). In the final analyses, it may be that elder mistreatment will be viewed as "unmet needs of the elderly," as inadequate care (Fulmer & O'Malley, 1987), or components of caregiver burden (Phillips, Rempusheski, & Morrison, 1989).

FIRST-WAVE STUDIES

The earliest studies on elder abuse were primarily exploratory descriptive survey studies with nonrandom samples (Block & Sinnott, 1979; Douglass, Hickey, & Noel, 1980; Lau & Kosberg, 1978; McLaughlin, Nickell, & Gill, 1980; O'Malley et al., 1978; Pepper & Oakar, 1981). The purpose of these studies was to examine the phenomenon of elder mistreatment and begin to provide information about its prevalence and nature. Within the context of these studies, theoretical frameworks were being liberally borrowed from the family violence arena, specifically from the child abuse literature. It was postulated that there is a causal relationship between dependency, nonnormal care providers, transgenerational violence, caregiver stress, and isolation of elders with elder mistreatment. O'Malley and associates used a mail survey approach to raise consciousness in the professional and paraprofessional realm related to elder mistreatment, and, with a 32% response rate ($N = 332$), found that most professionals reported some sort of abuse with physical abuse accounting for 41% of injuries. In that study, victims were reported as likely to be older (over 75 years), female (80%), and to have some sort of physical or mental disability (75%). Most of the abuse occurred at the hands of relatives. The Lau and Kosberg study (1978) looked at the prevalence of elder mistreatment prior to admission in a chronic illness center consisting of 404 retrospective chart reviews. This study reported 77% of abuse in women, with 82% of the abusers being relatives of victims, and physical abuse constituting the largest category (75%). Block and Sinott (1979) used a three-part inferential survey with a relatively low response rate in order to glean 26 cases of elder mistreatment. A retrospective case analysis was conducted from public agencies and the findings revealed victims to be older, female (81%), with psychological abuse (name calling, verbal threats, bullying) noted to be the most common (58%), with physical abuse (hitting, kicking) at 38% and material abuse (misuse of money or goods)at 46%. Douglass et al. (1980) used a convenience sample of 228 professionals in five communities and a semistructured interview in order to learn about types of mistreatment. In that study, passive neglect was the most prevalent type of abuse and due to the nonprobability, nonrandom sample, little else could be determined from the data. In the McLaughlin et al. (1980) study, a convenience sample of 31 telephone interviews and 51 questionnaires gleaned a 4.5% prevalence rate of elder abuse. This study noted that most abused elders were female, over the age of 75, and functionally disabled. Abusers were noted to be relatives of the victim and there seemed to be family stress involved. The Pepper and Oakar (1981) study used an exploratory survey, sending question-naires to all state human service departments, chiefs of police, visiting nurse associations, and interviews with experts. Although a nonrandom sample, they reported from their data that the typical abused elder was a dependent woman over 75 years of age and that the typical abuser was a male caretaker under great stress. The report stated that over one million elders might be abuse vic-tims and that physical violence was the most common form, followed by financial and psychologic abuse. The pattern in these early studies suggested that the utilization of nonrandom, convenience samples for the purpose of glean-ing exploratory information did much to raise the social consciousness related to elder mistreatment but little to advance the science of elder mistreatment.

SECOND-WAVE STUDIES

Following these first-wave studies, a series of papers criticized early work and spawned studies aimed at correcting previous criticisms. In the early 1980s, it became clear that clinicians were joining the social scientists in delving into the problem of elder mistreatment. O'Malley, Everitt, O'Malley and Campion (1983) published a seminal article in the *Annals of Internal Medicine* that alerted physicians to the possibility of elder mistreatment and their responsibility for detection and prevention. Although the initial article was not databased, those researchers went on to conduct a study of 22 cases of elder abuse and neglect in order to define categories of caretaker-mediated inadequate care (O'Malley, O'Malley, Everitt, & Sarson, 1984). Using a nonrandom convenience sample, 22 cases of family abuse or neglect were reviewed by a physician and nurse, one or both of whom were involved in the subject's care. The OARS Multidi-mensional Functional Assessment Questionnaire was adapted for use in review-ing the medical and social service records of these subjects. Cases were divided into three categories on the basis of the subject's score on the activities of daily living (ADL/IADL) instrumental activities of daily living section and the num-ber and severity of the subject's current medical problems. The authors sug-gested that three categories of caretaker-mediated inadequate care can be defined. Category I involved subjects who were extremely impaired, with multiple care needs; category II indicated subjects with significant care needs that could only be completely met with the assistance of the caretaker, and category III cases were clearly abusive as they concerned cases of extortion of money, threats of violence, or violence due to alcohol. The authors suggested that category III cases require a very different intervention from categories I and II, which really reflect "unmet needs."

Hudson, Johnson, and O'Brien (1986) conducted a health-care provider survey using a statewide survey of Michigan and North Carolina health care providers in order to determine the knowledge related to resources necessary for effective identification and intervention of elder mistreatment. The random sample included 3001 primary care physicians and nurse practitioners from those states. Through mail questionnaires they collected information related to six categories of elder mistreatment (physical, psychological, self-abuse, exploitation, neglect, and abandonment). Forty-seven questions, six of which were open-ended, were used. A response rate of 33.6% was reported, and of the 731 respondents with elderly clients, 361 (49.4%) reported they had never had a case of elder mistreatment. Three hundred and seventy respondents reported an elder mistreatment case accounting for approximately a third of the returned surveys. Chi-square analyses were used to compare the elder abuse experience variable with other selected variables. Results indicated that the economic status of the elder and home visits by the primary care professional were significantly related to answering "yes" to an elder mistreatment experience. Also, those professionals who rated elder abuse as important and pervasive were more likely to report an event.

In that same year, Hudson and Johnson (1986) published a review of the literature and provided an analysis and summary of 31 studies. They concluded that most of the work to that point, which was through 1985, was exploratory and descriptive. Most of the published research consisted of exploratory mail surveys about the nature and extent of elder mistreatment, instrumentation work, or efforts related to definitional problems in the field. The role of caregiver stress, functional decline, psychopathology of the caregiver, and violence patterns preexisting in the family were recurrent themes although there were virtually no theory development efforts to support them. At that point little was known concerning interventions to prevent or stop elder mistreatment.

PROGRAMS OF RESEARCH

Since the mid-1980s, a growing number of investigators with programs of research related to elder mistreatment have gone beyond the descriptive, exploratory surveys. In particular, the research programs of Phillips at the University of Arizona, Fulmer at Columbia University, and Pillemer at Cornell University have improved the science and understanding of elder mistreatment in a notable way. Although these three researchers have made significant contributions to the understanding of elder abuse they are not alone. Many researchers have now undertaken the investigation of this problem.

Clinical Programs and Clinically Focused Research

Phillips (1983), using an ex post factor correlational descriptive design with a purposive sample of 74 elderly, reported that demographic characteristics and certain theoretical variables such as anger, hostility, and stress were similar between groups labeled as "having a good relationship" or "an abusive neglectful relationship" related to their caregivers (Phillips, 1983). Using multiple regression analysis, a total of four causal models were tested using anger, depression, anxiety, and abuse as terminal dependent variables. The amount of explained variance ranged from 22% for anxiety to 58% for abuse. These data showed no significant difference in physical functioning between the abuse group and the good relationship group and noted that social isolation of the elder was an important causal variable in abuse. Phillips summarized her paper by stating that elder abuse is probably caused by the interaction of a number of key variables related to complex relationships. This study (Phillips, 1983) set the stage for her research, which led to the publication of a decision-making model for diagnosing and intervening in elder abuse and neglect (Phillips & Rempusheski, 1985). This model, generated from data obtained by tape-recorded interviews of 29 health care providers set forth categories and structural factors related to decision making about the use of the elder abuse/neglect label. Set A Categories were said to be those that defined the nature of the situation, whereas Set B Categories were those assessed to understand the reasons for the situation. A diagram of an empirically generated model published with those data reflected a path for decision making. In a companion paper, Phillips and Rempusheski (1986a), reported that four general themes can be noted in the interviews: (a) the abuser's or caregiver's acts, (b) the differentiation between abuse and neglect as related to the severity of the outcomes for the elder, (c) the intentionality of the act, and (d) the notion that abuse and neglect are closely related. The authors proposed that these four themes form the "conceptual underpinnings of decisions about who is and who is not abused or neglected."

The next phase of Phillips' research was focused upon family caregivers' perceptions of home care for frail elders (Phillips & Rempusheski, 1986b). Using the grounded-theory approach with 39 family caregivers, a theoretical model was generated to describe the dynamics of good quality and poor quality family caregiving, the relationships between selected contextual and perceptual variables and the behaviors exchanged between the dyad, and points at which interventions by nurses could be effective. This approach generated a model consisting of five constructs (personal identity of the elder, image of caregiving, caregiver's role beliefs, caregiver's behavioral strategies, and perceptions) and two related driving forces (currently salient role form and role interdependence). According to the developers, this model provides a partial explanation for the quality of family caregiving and an explanation for the phenomenon of elder abuse. The model, although theoretically instructive, has little clinical utility due to its complexity.

Moving from a qualitative to a quantitative approach, Phillips, Morrison, and Chae (1990a, 1990b) published the QUALCARE Scale, an instrument intended to measure the quality of homecare, which has been extensively tested for appropriate psychometric properties. Building on earlier work related to "Beliefs about Caregiving" (Phillips et al., 1989), the QUALCARE Scale has an interrater reliability percentage of agreement above the 0.70 criterion level, with evidence of appropriate internal consistency, criterion validity, and construct validity. This 53-item scale is in a Likert-type format and sets the stage for uniform assessment related to quality caregiving and elder mistreatment. Only recently available, it remains to be seen what the impact of the QUALCARE Scale will be on assessment for elder mistreatment. The QUALCARE Scale study seems to imply a standard of care that was unrealistic in the real world. For example, poor care is implied if the house is not neat. This may be an erroneous association, and thus brings the instrument's validity into question.

Fulmer and Ashley (1986) identified neglect as the most difficult and yet most prevalent form of mistreatment reported to protective service workers. Neglect is a particularly difficult phenomenon to investigate in the elderly due to the confounds of illness symptoms, normal age-related changes, and the pervasive ageism in our culture that precludes a thorough history and physical examination in elders, attributing clinical indicators as related to "old age." Earlier work by Fulmer and colleagues at the Beth Israel Hospital in Boston included neglect as a subset of abuse (Fulmer & Cahill, 1984). This proved to be problematic and led to efforts related to instrument development for elder mistreatment with specific attention to abuse, neglect, exploitation, and medical mistreatment (Fulmer, Street, & Carr, 1984). Follow-up psychometric testing on a larger sample ($N = 107$) led to the development of the Elder Assessment Instrument (EAI) with an interrater reliability of .83 and a content validity of .84 (Fulmer & O'Malley, 1987).

Further effort was made to examine clinical indicators of neglect by conducting an exploratory factor analysis to test the construct validity of items on the EAI specifically related to neglect. Those 15 items, selected by an expert panel, were included in a factor analysis in which the sample size was dropped to an unacceptably low level due to standard list-wise deletion procedures. An acceptable alternative chosen for this study was to eliminate those items with missing data on over 20% of the observations. Therefore, 9 of the original 15 items were available for factor analysis. The resultant Chronbach's alpha reliability for this nine-item index was .76. A factor analysis using orthogonal rotation revealed that these nine neglect indicators clustered in three catagories: nutrition/hydration, skin integrity, and elimination. It seems then that the EAI identifies the need for careful assessment that relates specifically to each of these areas.

Recently, investigators at Yale-New Haven Hospital reviewed 3153 cases of individuals over 65 presenting at an emergency unit (EU) (Fulmer, McMahon, Baer-Hines, & Forget, 1992). This study was preceded by an intensive training period for all staff nurses in that unit. A nurse specialist with expertise in elder mistreatment reviewed the registration sheet and EU record of every elder over 65. Using a purposive, nonrandom sample of 3153 consecutive charts, 4% ($N = 127$) indicated some form of elder mistreatment (abuse, neglect, violence, exploitation, or abandonment). The most prevalent form was neglect ($N = 70$), followed by abuse ($N = 43$), violent crime ($N = 8$), abandonment ($N = 4$), and exploitation ($N = 1$). Associations with mistreatment included the status of being unmarried, nonwhite, without insurance, or with a documentation of dementia or delirium. This would suggest that vulnerable individuals, by virtue of lower socioeconomic status or cognitive decline, are most at risk. The limitations of this study include the use of only one site for data collection, the nonrandom sample, and the use of emergency unit records to document cognitive status instead of a clinical diagnostic screen (such as the Mini-Mental State Examination).

Ferguson and Beck (1983) have also contributed to the clinical assessment literature and provided the H.A.L.F. tool for assessing elder mistreatment. This acronym refers to the assessment of health status, attitudes toward aging, living arrangements, and finances. Practical in length and easy to use, the major drawback is that no psychometric testing has been reported. Similarly, Hamilton (1989) has published the REAH tool (Risk of Elder Abuse in the Home), which can be scored from 0 to 15 and looks at the vulnerability of the elder as well as the stress in the situation. Content validity has been established by an expert panel ($N = 10$) using a range of 1 to 5 (least important to most important), dropping scores below 3.

It is clear that clinicians have an important role to play in the evaluation of elder mistreatment. In one study (Daniels, Baumhover, & Clark-Daniels, 1989) conducted in Alabama, a stratified random sample of physicians likely to be in regular contact with elderly patients was conducted. A total of 176 questionnaires were returned for a 46% response rate. The questionnaire contained demographic items, physician-generated profiles of typical abused or neglected persons, questions concerning physicians' alertness to elder abuse cases, and questions regarding their knowledge of Alabama law. The results were mixed with regard to the definition and diagnosis of elder mistreatment. Over 60% of the respondents believed that an experienced physician could accurately diagnose cases of abuse. Yet 77% expressed doubt or uncertainty about the availability of clear-cut definitions from the American Medical Association. The majority of physicians responded that most incidents of abuse involve minor, nonreportable injuries, and 58% of the physicians responding reported seeing abuse in their practice. It is important to note that since that paper the American Medical Association (1992) has developed a set of guidelines for detecting elder abuse.

From a different perspective, Dolan and Blakely (1989) analyzed data from 1,137 adult protective service workers in 40 states and Washington, DC. They reported that nearly all respondents had come in contact with at least one case of elder abuse or neglect during the preceding year. This makes sense, given that the usual mechanism for reporting involves a professional report to a state agency that refers to a protective service worker. In that light, it may be that protective service workers need a more efficient mechanism for feedback to the physician related to elder abuse cases in order to help clinicians be more vigilant regarding repeat cases. In another survey of state public health departments and procedures for reporting elder abuse (Ehrlich & Anetzberger, 1991), a mail questionnaire was sent to all 50 states with a 94% response. The results demonstrated an inverse relationship between awareness of the laws and regulations of specific activities to support the reporting process. Ninety-four percent of respondents were aware of the state laws but only 20% to 28% reported the use of written procedures for training materials specifically designed for health personnel. This would suggest that there are few support systems in the clinical arena to guide clinicians in reporting elder mistreatment. Limitations of mail surveys include the possibility of a nonrepresentative sample and misinterpretation of items. Further, it is unclear whether the person answering the survey was, in fact, the most appropriate person to respond.

Social Science Programs

Pillemer, a sociologist who has been conducting research on elder abuse and mistreatment since the early 1980s, also has contributed to science in the field. His early collaborative work with Wolf and Godkin, (Wolf, Godkin, & Pillemer, 1984) in a 3-year demonstration project that described three model projects compared abuse cases with randomly selected nonabuse cases in the Worcester site and described the perpetrators as more likely to be male and the victims to be living in households with family members. Victims and nonabused clients were similar in age, gender, and health status. Both victims and perpetrators were found to have more problems with psychological and emotional health, including alcohol abuse, than those who were not abused. Cases were next analyzed by type of mistreatment, and to the extent possible, comment was made regarding differences across the types. Psychopathology of the abuser was strongly supported, whereas dependency of the elder was not. In fact, these researchers argued that it was the dependency of the caregiver on the elder that was the more likely pattern. Stress and isolation were reported as having "lesser influence" and were said to exacerbate rather than cause elder mistreatment. No statement could be made relative to the "cycle of family violence" theory. This study was carefully designed and is one of the most frequently referenced papers on the subject.

This work was followed by an examination of social isolation and elder mistreatment (Pillemer, 1985) using the Three Model Project data. Focusing on one type of mistreatment, that of physical abuse, the study used direct interviews with clients and included a matched control group of nonabused elders. The sample consisted of 42 physically abused elders and 42 nonabused controls. All interviews were conducted by the same interviewer. The researchers suggested social support to be a moderator of life stress and the presence of an outside person to serve as a deterrent to mistreatment. This gives rise to the notion that an outside person can be a strategy for the prevention of mistreatment, but the author is quick to caution that more studies are needed to confirm this finding.

Pillemer is probably best known for his work on a random sample survey on the prevalence of elder abuse (Pillemer & Finkelhor, 1989) because it was the first large-scale random sample survey of elder abuse and neglect. Interviews were conducted with 2020 community-dwelling elders in a large northeastern metropolitan area in order to ascertain the prevalence of certain types of mistreatment including physical violence, verbal aggression, and neglect. The prevalence rate reported for these phenomena was 32 per 1000, and spouses were found to be the most likely abusers. Both men and women were almost as likely to be victims. This was the first time that spouses could be documented as the likely perpetrators, which led others to comment that elder abuse was simply domestic violence "grown old," but others challenged the use of proxies for elders in the sample who were cognitively impaired. Others also challenged the methodology despite the authors' explanation for the process. The finding that men are as likely to be victims as women has also been questioned and warrants further review. This study has been cited widely for prevalence estimates on elder mistreatment, however.

Success in shedding new light on the prevalence of elder mistreatment in the community next led Pillemer and Moore (1989) to look at abuse of patients in nursing homes. A random sample survey was conducted of 577 nurses and nursing aides employed in long-term care facilities in New Hampshire. Every effort was made to ensure a representative sample of nursing homes and hence, a representative sample of respondents. Of the 577 respondents, 61% were nursing aides, 20% were licensed practical nurses, and 19% were registered nurses. Demographics on the sample were reported along with information on the employment history. Questionnaires were based on the Conflict Tactics Scale (CTS), a widely accepted instrument in the family violence research field (Straus, 1979). Thirty-six percent of the sample had seen at least one incident of physical abuse in the preceding year, with the most frequent type of physical abuse noted as excessive restraint. The second most frequent type of abuse observed included pushing, grabbing, shoving, or pinching a patient. Slapping or hitting was reported at 12%. Eighty-one percent of respondents observed at least one psychologically abusive incident in the preceding year, with the most frequent type reported as yelling, with over 50% reporting that they observed someone swearing at a patient. This is the first large-scale study to provide data on elder mistreatment in long-term care facilities and has generated much discussion.

Pillemer and Finkelhor (1989) examined the belief that abuse results from burden and stress, using elder abuse victims and a nonabused control group. These data suggested that the elder is a functionally intact person who is victimized by ill and socioemotionally unstable relatives. The authors concluded that as in other areas of family violence research, abuser characteristics tend to be more powerful predictors than the victim characteristics. This supports the theory of the psychopathology of the abuser as a causative factor in elder mistreatment. A recent study by Pillemer and Suitor (1992) has focused on violence and violent feelings, and explores the important difference between the two states. Spousal relationships, advanced age, and self-esteem were reported as significantly different in those who fear becoming violent versus those who do not have that fear. In terms of the difference between the fear of violence group and the actual violence group, only violence by the care recipient ($p < .05$) and spousal relationship to the care recipient ($p < .006$) were significant. The authors noted the need for longitudinal studies in order to discern any patterns in the escalation of violence over the period of a caregiving relationship. None of the work of Pillemer and colleagues has specifically focused on neglect as a form of elder mistreatment, but instead, tend to use only the CTS, which is a limitation. This research serves as the highest quality knowledge base in the field today, however. Specific studies that methodically address the major theories for why elder mistreatment occurs must be conducted in large random samples with multicultural representation.

SUMMARY AND FUTURE RESEARCH DIRECTIONS

In conclusion, it is fair to say that the elder mistreatment literature has grown in sophistication, substance, and volume over the past 15 years. Early work, which created a societal recognition of the problem, has now led to research that seems to be clustered in three groups: surveys of awareness and practice, instrumentation, and case-control studies. Future clinical and social science research needs to focus heavily on intervention studies for the prevention of the various types of elder mistreatment, based on a sound understanding of high-risk individuals. Longitudinal studies of elders at risk are also key to determining predisposition and obtaining accurate incidence rates. Finally, far more quantitative studies that enable researchers to hear the stories of elders who have been mistreated should be conducted. The next 15 years of research have the opportunity to stem the tide of a potential elder mistreatment epidemic based on current estimates of the scope of the problem and the demographics of America.

REFERENCES

American Medical Association. (1992). *Diagnostic and treatment guidelines on elderly abuse and neglect.* Chicago: Author.

Block, M., & Sinnott, J. (Eds.). (1979). *The battered elderly syndrome: An exploratory study.* College Park, MD: University of Maryland, Center on Aging.

Callahan, J. J. (1986). Editors perspective. *Pride Institute Journal of Long-term Home Health Care, 5*(5), 2.

Callahan, J. J. (1988). Elder abuse: Some questions for policy makers. *The Gerontologist, 28,* 453–458.

Daniels, S. R., Baumhover, L. A., & Clark-Daniels, C. L. (1989). Physician's mandatory reporting of elder abuse. *The Gerontologist, 29,* 321–327.

Dolon, R., & Blakely, B. (1989). Elder abuse and neglect: A study of adult protective service workers in the United States. *Journal of Elder Abuse and Neglect, 1*(3), 31–49.

Douglass, R. L., & Hickey, T.(1981). Neglect and abuse of older family member: Professionals' perspectives and case experiences. *The Gerontologist, 21,* 171–176.

Douglass, R. L., Hickey, T., & Noel, M. (1980). *Elder abuse.* Ann Arbor: University of Michigan Press.

Ehrlich, P., & Anetzberger, G. (1991). Survey of state public health department on procedures for reporting elder abuse. *Public Health Reports, 106,* 151–154.

Ferguson, D., & Beck, C. (1983). H.A.L.F.—A tool to assess elder abuse within the family. *Geriatric Nursing, 4,* 301–304.

Fulmer, T., & Ashley, J. (1986). Neglect: What part of abuse? *Pride Institute Journal of Long Term Home Health Care, 5*(4), 18–24.

Fulmer, T., & Cahill, V. (1984). Assessing elder abuse: A study. *Journal of Gerontological Nursing, 10*(12), 16–20.

Fulmer, T., McMahon, D., Baer-Hines, M., & Forget, B. (1992). Prevalence of abuse, neglect, abandonment, violence and exploitation: An analysis of all elderly patients seen in one emergency department over a six-month period. *Journal of Emergency Nursing, 18,* 505–510.

Fulmer, T., & O'Malley T. (1987). *Inadequate care of the elderly: A health care perspective on abuse and neglect.* New York: Springer Publishing Co.

Fulmer, T., Street, S., & Carr, K. (1984). Abuse of the elderly: Screening and detection. *Journal of Emergency Nursing, 10,* 131–140.

Hamilton, G. P. (1989). Using a prevent elder abuse family systems approach. *Journal of Gerontological Nursing, 15*(3), 21–26.

Hudson, M. F., & Johnson, T. F. (1986). Elder neglect and abuse: A review of the literature. In C. Eisdorfer (Ed.), *Annual Review of Geriatrics and Gerontology* (pp. 81–134). New York: Springer Publishing Co.

Hudson, M. F., Johnson, T. F., & O'Brien, J. (1986). *Report of the Health Care Provider Survey on Elder Abuse: The experiences of primary care physicians and nurse practitioners in Michigan and North Carolina.* Unpublished manuscript.

Lau, E., & Kosberg, J. (1978). Abuse of the elderly by informal care providers. *Aging, 22*(9), 5–10.

McLaughlin, J. S., Nickell, J. P., & Gill, L. (1980, June 11). U.S. House of Representatives. Select Committee on Aging. An epidemiological investigation of elderly abuse in southern Maine and New Hampshire. In *Elder abuse* (pp. 111–147) (Publication No. 68-463). Washington, DC: U.S. Government Printing Office.

O'Malley, H. C., Segars, H., Perez, R., Mitchell, V., & Knuepel, G. M. (1978). *Elder abuse in Massachusetts: A survey of professionals and paraprofessionals.* Boston: Boston Legal Research and Services for the Elderly.

O'Malley T.A., Everitt, D., O'Malley H., & Campion, E. (1983). Identifying and preventing family-mediated abuse and neglect of elderly persons. *Annals of Internal Medicine, 98,* 998–1005.

O'Malley, T. A., O'Malley, H. C., Everitt, D. A., & Sarson, D. (1984). Categories of family-mediated abuse and neglect of elderly persons. *Journal of the American Geriatric Society, 32,* 362–369.

Pepper, C., & Oakar, M. R. (1981). U.S. House of Representatives Select Committee on Aging. In *Elder abuse: An examination of a hidden problem.* (Publication No. 97-277). Washington, DC: U.S. Government Printing Office.

Phillips, L. R. (1983). Abuse and Neglect of the Frail elderly at home: An exploration of theoretical relationships. *Journal of Advanced Nursing, 8,* 379–392.

Phillips, L. R., Morrison, E. F., & Chae, Y. M. (1990a). The QUALCARE Scale: Developing an instrument to measure quality of homecare. *International Journal of Nursing Studies, 27*(1), 61–75.

Phillips, L. R., Morrison, E. F., & Chae, Y. M. (1990b). The QUALCARE Scale: Testing of a measurement instrument for clinical practice. *International Journal of Nursing Studies, 27*(1), 77–91.

Phillips, L. R., & Rempusheski, V. F. (1985). A decision making model for diagnosing and intervening in elder abuse and neglect. *Nursing Research, 34,* 134–140.

Phillips, L. R., & Rempusheski, V. F. (1986a). Making decisions about elder abuse. Social Casework. *The Journal of Contemporary Social Work, 67,* 131–140.

Phillips, L. R., & Rempusheski, V. F. (1986b). Caring for the frail elderly at home: Toward a theoretical explanation of the dynamics of poor quality family caregiving. *Advances in Nursing Science, 8*(4), 62–84.

Phillips, L. R., Rempusheski, V. F., & Morrison, E. (1989). Developing and testing the Beliefs about Caregiving Scale. *Research in Nursing & Health, 12,* 207–220.

Pillemer, K. A. (1985, Fall). Social isolation and elder abuse. *Response,* 2–4.

Pillemer, K.A., & Finkelhor, D. (1988). The prevalence of elder abuse: A random sample. *The Gerontologist, 28*(1), 51–57.

Pillemer, K. A., & Finkelhor, D. (1989). Causes of elder abuse: Caregiver stress versus problem relatives. *American Journal of Orthopsychiatry, 59,* 179–187.

Pillemer, K. A., & Moore, D. W. (1989). Abuse of patients in nursing homes: Findings from a survey of staff. *The Gerontologist, 29,* 314–320.

Pillemer, K. A., & Suitor, J. J. (1992). Violence and violent feelings: What causes them among family caregivers? *Journal of Gerontology, 47,* S165–S172.

Quinn, M. J., & Tomita, S. K. (1986). *Elder abuse and neglect: Causes, diagnosis and intervention strategies.* New York: Springer Publishing Co.

Straus, M. A. (1979). Measuring intrafamily conflict and violence: The Conflict Tactics Scale (CTS). *Journal of Marriage and Family, 41,* 75–88.

Wolf, R. S., Godkin, M. A., & Pillemer, K. A. (1984). Elder abuse and neglect: Findings from three model projects. Worcester: University of Massachusetts Medical Center, University Center on Aging.

Chapter 4

Rural Health and Health-Seeking Behaviors

CLARANN WEINERT, S.C.
COLLEGE OF NURSING
MONTANA STATE UNIVERSITY

MARY E. BURMAN
SCHOOL OF NURSING
UNIVERSITY OF WYOMING

CONTENTS

Rural America holds a sense of charm and nostalgia. For some, it is a place where for generations their families have engaged in farming, ranching, mining, or logging. For others, rural America provides an escape from urban tensions; a place of recreation, relaxation, or retirement. Rural can mean "a place to get away from" for some people and for others, a "place to get away to" (Lee, 1991a, p. 7).

Rural America can probably best be described with the paradox of stability with change. Currently, 77% of the nation's counties are classified as nonmetropolitan and nearly 15,000 towns have a population of less that 2500 (U.S. Department of Health and Human Services, 1993). The number of people living in rural America has increased over the last 40 years from 54 million in 1950 to 62 million in 1990, with 7.7 million older Americans living in rural areas.

Cordes (1985) warned that it is a serious flaw to equate agriculture with rurality. The rural nonfarm population outnumbers the rural farm population by about seven to one. Today, with advanced agricultural technology, food can be provided for the whole country by only 2% of the population (Wright, 1993). The rural economy is diversified, including manufacturing, national parks, recreational services, and retirement communities and is a major factor in the overall United States economy.

Regional variation, manifested by rural poor in the South, Hispanic rural dwellers in the Southwest, and farmers and ranchers of the West and Great Plains, is longstanding. This diversity is further heightened by small rural enclaves such as the Pennsylvania Amish, the California Filipinos, and the Vietnamese in Texas. Changing sociocultural and demographic profiles and geographic contrasts present major challenges in rural definition and research focusing on health and health care delivery.

RESEARCH CHARACTERISTICS

Research Methods

Rural research consists of widely differing levels of sophistication, often divergent in content and conclusions, and ranges from highly structured data-based studies to individual case studies and anecdotal reports. Information sources vary from federal publications to narrower regional publications to scientific reports in research and other professional journals. Consequently, literature is not always readily accessible, as publication may be in obscure and difficult-to-access places.

This chapter is focused on health status, health perceptions and beliefs, and health-seeking behaviors of rural residents. The review does not include articles on the following rural topics: health care delivery, health care personnel recruitment and retention, or education of nurses or other health care providers. The priorities of this review are based on the premise that in order to understand health care delivery in rural areas, the rural context must be understood. In addition, much of rural health care literature is not research-based. In the face of health care reform, the temptation is to focus specifically on health care delivery in rural areas. Nurses who practice in rural settings and those responsible for health care policy and planning are obliged to have a good understanding of rural dwellers and their environment in order to undertake relevant research and provide appropriate and cost effective services.

Research articles were located through computer and manual searches of Index Medicus, Cumulative Index of Nursing and Allied Health Literature, and Sociological Abstracts. The last three years of *Nursing Research, Research in Nursing and Health, Western Journal of Nursing, Journal of Rural Health*, and *Rural Sociology* were manually searched (1990–1993). In addition, a survey of active rural nurse researchers was conducted requesting input regarding the direction of rural nursing research and soliciting bibliographic information. Only research conducted on United States rural populations and published from 1983 to the present is reported in this chapter. Unpublished research was included when obtained. Classic literature and literature reviews also are cited to provide background for recent research.

Rural Research Themes

Four major types of rural health care research were found. First, a number of researchers specifically examined rural and urban differences. Second, many investigators examined health and health-related phenomena in a rural area. Third, the focus of many of the articles was on a concept such as chronic illness; in such cases, rurality was examined as one of several demographic variables. Finally, typical "rural" populations, such as farm workers, migrants, and Native Americans, were investigated.

DEFINITION OF RURAL

The conceptualization and operationalization of rural remains problematic and is evident in the research reviewed for this chapter. There are two widely used definitions. First, the United States Census Bureau (1987) designates those living in towns of 2500 or more as urban. Those not classified as urban are considered rural. Second, the Office of Management and Budget (1983) differentiates metropolitan from nonmetropolitan residents based on Metropolitan Statistical Areas (MSA). An MSA is a city of 50,000 or more residents, or an urbanized area with at least 50,000 that is part of a county or counties with at least 100,000 people.

Hewitt (1992) noted that conclusions about health can be substantively different when using these two definitions. For example, the elderly make up a larger proportion of the total population in nonmetropolitan, compared to metropolitan areas. If the urban/rural categorization is used the opposite is true, however; the proportion of elderly is greater in urban areas than in rural areas (Hewitt, 1992). Consequently, changing lifestyles, migration patterns, and sociocultural factors can be blurred by using one of these definitions without specifying its limitations (Cordes, 1989; Hassinger, 1982; Hewitt, 1992; Ide, 1992; Lee, 1991a).

Other conceptualizations of rural have been proposed. The National Rural Health Association suggested the designation of frontier, defined as less than six persons per square mile, to be a finer delineation of rurality. Urbanized rural counties are defined further as those with population of 25,000 or more and not adjacent to an MSA. Counties can meet both criteria (Hewitt, 1992), however. Jordan and Hargrove (1987) developed an eight-category definition. Weinert and Boik (1993) proposed a relative measure of rurality, the Montana State University (MSU) Rurality Index, which can be used to assign a degree of rurality that has within study specificity using only two variables: miles to emergency care and the population of the county. This measure may provide a sensitive and valid measure for researchers to distinguish the degree of rurality for a given population.

Conceptual and measurement issues are not trivial and give rise to serious problems in evaluating and interpreting research. On one level, "rural" merely describes a place of residence. Consequently, differences between urban and rural areas would be expected to be minimal. Rurality also may reflect sociocultural differences and rural areas then would be distinct from urban areas. The challenge for researchers is to identify aspects of rurality that affect health and health care and to avoid exploring rurality merely for rurality sake.

HEALTH

Health Beliefs

Health Perceptions.   Rural and urban dwellers may perceive health differently and certain views of health may be more prevalent among rural dwellers (Long, 1993). In ethnographic interviews, rural dwellers defined health as the ability to work (Weinert & Long, 1987). Ross (1982) and Lee (1989) reported that rural persons were more likely than urban dwellers to associate health with the ability to work, function, and perform daily tasks. Older adults defined health as being able to do what one wanted to or needed to do, and for some, health meant not having any pain (Davis et al., 1991). Brown (1990) found that health was viewed as "connected independence" and was defined as being able to do what needed to be done, implying independence. Yet, in order to remain healthy, elders needed to "stay in the world" or be connected. The value placed on independence and self-reliance also was found in several other studies (Counts & Boyle, 1987; Thorson & Powell, 1992). A central element in the definition of health for rural dwellers in different regions of the country is the ability to work. Long and Weinert (1992) found that for individuals with a chronic illness, place of residence may not be an important variable in determining how persons described their own health or how they defined what it means to be healthy.

Bigbee (1991) noted that hardiness fits well with the independence, self-reliance, and self-care found in rural areas. Urban families were hardier than rural families (Dunkin, Holzwart, & Stratton, 1993), however. Hardiness, dignity, privacy, self-sufficiency, and independence contributed to the competence of older rural adults, but also may have led to delays in seeking health care (Lee, 1993).

Attitudes Toward Stigmatized Conditions.   Rural residents have been thought to hold more negative attitudes regarding mental illness and, consequently, those with mental illness suffer more stigma. Rural residents in the Midwest had positive attitudes about mental illness (Flaskerud & Kviz, 1983), however. Rost, Smith, and Taylor (1993) found no differences between urban and rural residents on labeling of persons seeking help for depression.

AIDS is another stigmatized disease. Older rural adolescents were more likely to express disapproval about persons with AIDS (Miller, Qualtere-Burcher, Labuer, Rockow, & Bauman, 1990). In addition, there were ethnic differences, with rural African Americans and Native Americans displaying less tolerance for persons with AIDS than rural whites and hispanics.

Physical and Mental Well-Being

Rural dwellers have been considered to be in poorer health than their urban counterparts. Given the diversity of rural America and that health is a relative term, however, the relationship between rurality and health is more complex than a simple linear relationship.

Children and Adolescents.   Relatively few researchers have examined the general well-being of rural children and adolescents; most have focused on specific health conditions or health behavior in children. McManus, Newacheck, and Weader (1990) found few differences in the health status of rural adolescents as compared to urban adolescents.

Adults.   The physical and mental well-being of adults and older adults has been the focus of most studies (Preston & Mansfield, 1991). In a national survey, physical health was perceived to be better by urban residents, whereas rural residents had stronger social health, for example, family interaction, organizational involvement, and social integration (Eggebeen & Lichter, 1993). Metropolitan and nonmetropolitan residents did not differ in well-being in another national study; health perceptions were more strongly related to financial status, marital status, and education (Mookherjee, 1992).

Rural residents perceived less worry, general pain, anxiety, and depression, but lower physical health than an urban comparison group (Long & Weinert, 1992; Weinert & Long, 1987). Urban families experienced more stressors than rural families (Marotz-Baden, 1988). Stressors differed, with rural families experiencing more economic stressors and urban families reporting more work and family stressors.

Rural poor had lower perceived health than urban poor (Amato & Zuo, 1992). Poor African Americans had lower psychological well-being in urban areas, whereas psychological well-being of poor whites was lower in rural areas.

Husbands' unemployment led to greater stress in wives than in the husbands themselves (Wilhelm & Ridley, 1988). Rural residents with more hardiness rated their mental and social health higher than those with less hardiness (Lee, 1991b). This did not hold true for physical health, however. Rural residents in stable marital relationships had fewer health problems than those in unstable relationships (Zvonkovic, Guss, & Ladd, 1988).

Farm Workers.   Yesalis, Lemke, Wallace, Kohourt, and Morris (1985) found few differences in health status based on farmwork history. Farm women had better physical functioning and experienced fewer general symptoms than nonfarm women. Older farmers and ranchers perceived their physical health less positively than younger farmers and ranchers (Lee, 1993). Their physical and mental health in general were no different than a comparison sample that included urban residents, however. In farm operators, stress was related to the amount of financial instability of farming (Belyea & Lobao, 1990; Geller, Bultena, & Lasley, 1988). Similarly, Duncan, Volk, and Lewis (1988) found that income adequacy and stability were related to well-being of farm wives and husbands. Farm men and women experienced a variety of symptoms, such as trouble concentrating and loss of appetite and nausea, that were related to farm stressors like financial worries, equipment problems, and personal illness (Heffernan & Heffernan, 1986; Weigel & Weigel, 1988). To further the understanding of stress, Ide and Arquistain (1993) have developed a scale to measure stress in rural farmers and ranchers.

Women.   Well-being of rural and urban women, measured as stress, life satisfaction, and exhaustion, did not differ significantly (Mansfield, Preston, & Crawford, 1988). Lifestyle factors, such as having young children at home and health status, were the strongest predictors of stress. Similarly, Bigbee (1988, 1990) found no differences in stress (number of stressful life events) and illness occurrence in rural and urban women. Rural women tended to perceive more environmentally related stressors, whereas urban women perceived more financially related stress (Bigbee, 1987). Integration of work and family roles was more important in the well-being of employed rural women than urban women (Walters & McHenry, 1985). Berkowitz and Perkins (1984), however, argued that interpersonal dynamics were a greater factor in stress of farm women than home and work roles.

Older Adults. The well-being of older rural adults has received the most attention. Scheidt (1984, 1986) developed well-being profiles of rural elderly and found that the majority were "partially engaged." They were physically and mentally healthy and active in the community, but did not have frequent social contacts. A smaller percentage were "disengaged," less healthy and socially involved, or "fully engaged," healthy and socially active. Only a small percentage were "frail," with little social support and poorer health. Similar clusters were found in a study of older adults by Preston and Mansfield (1984). In another study, rural "old-old" (aged 75+) were as mentally and physically healthy as those 60 to 74 years of age (Halpert & Zimmerman, 1986). McCulloch (1991) examined a cohort of rural women in 1976 and 1986. Ten-year survivors had higher educational levels and were more likely to be married and to have rated their health as good at time one. Quevillon and Lee (1983) found that the well-being of institutionalized rural elders was related to quality, not quantity, of social interaction. In noninstitutionalized rural elderly, morale was related to availability of a confidante, shopping enjoyment, neighbor and community satisfaction, and fulfillment of transportation needs (McGhee, 1984).

In another cluster of studies, comparisons of well-being were made between urban and rural older adults. Using several different measures, well-being did not differ between rural and urban elderly (Kivett, 1985). Health dependency did not differ significantly between urban and rural residents (Krout, 1989). Coward and Cutler (1988) found that older farm residents had fewer functional limitations, whereas nonmetropolitan, nonfarm residents had more functional limitations. These findings in several states were congruent with findings from a study done on the national level (Cutler & Coward, 1988). Older adults in metropolitan communities reported more stress than those in nonmetropolitan communities (Preston & Crawford, 1990). Moreover, Dwyer and Miller (1990) examined stress in caregivers and care-receivers in urban, small city, and rural areas and found differences by place of residence as well as age, functional ability, and ethnic background.

Specific Health Conditions

Occupational, demographic, and sociocultural factors in rural areas may predispose individuals to specific health conditions. For example, some rural areas have higher proportions of older adults, leading to higher rates of chronic illness.

Infant Mortality. Baker and Kotelchuck (1989) compared birthweight-specific infant mortality between an urban area and a rural area. Both blacks and whites in rural areas had higher infant mortality rates at all birthweights. Zadinsky and Boettcher (1992) examined the preventability of infant mortality in rural areas. Interestingly, nurses and physicians differed in their perception of preventability; the nurses believed the deaths were preventable, the physicians did not.

Infectious Diseases.   The incidence of viral respiratory diseases did not differ between urban and rural children (Belshe, Van Voris & Mufson, 1983). Adams and Perkin (1985) found high rates of intestinal parasitic diseases in rural children, however. Susceptibility to rubella infection has declined in a rural area (Crowder, Higgins & Frost, 1987). Several investigators found that tuberculosis was a problem in rural areas (Gross, Silverman, Bloch, Smith, & Rogers, 1989; Robinson & Comstock, 1992). HIV prevalence was lower in rural than urban practice settings (Calonge, Petersen, Miller, & Marshall, 1993). Influenza/pneumonia mortality rates were found to be higher in rural areas in comparison with urban areas (Schorr, Crabtree, Wagner, & Wetterau, 1989).

Accidents and Occupational Hazards.   Farm accidents and other rural occupational health hazards have received considerable attention by researchers. In general, mortality due to accidents is higher in rural than urban areas (Schorr et al., 1989). In addition, fatal farm accident rates were higher for boys than for girls (Salmi et al., 1989; Stallones, 1989). Geller, Ludtke, and Stratton (1990) attributed farm accidents in adults to the financial instability of farming. They noted a discernible pattern in which high-risk operators tended to be younger and have a higher debt-to-asset ratio. The findings lend support to their hypothesis that financially distressed farmers are more likely to experience a farm accident.

Adults with a history of farm work and residence in predominantly agricultural counties had higher rates of glioblastoma multiform (Smith-Rooker, Garrett, Hodges, & Shue, 1992). Older men with a history of farm work had a lower prevalence of Parkinson's disease and prostate conditions, but higher rates of respiratory disease (Yesalie et al., 1985). Farmers, despite having lower incomes, less education, and less preventive care, had lower mean blood pressure than persons in other occupations (Gold & Franks, 1989). Pratt (1990) conducted a thorough review of occupational health problems related to farming as well as mining and logging in rural areas. Farm workers were affected by psychological illness, injuries, parasites, skin disease, and the dangers of agrichemicals. Farmers faced the hazards of stress and had a high suicide rate and job-related fatality rate. Miners and loggers worked in dangerous environments and suffered from acute and chronic problems: trauma, respiratory illness, vascular problems, and malignancy.

Chronic Physical Problems.   Edentulism rates were lower in rural areas than in the older population in general (Hunt, Beck, Lemke, Kohout, & Wallace, 1985). The incidence and impact of low back pain in rural areas was substantial (Lavsky-Shulan et al., 1985), however.

Morbidity and mortality rates have been a common measure of chronic illness and a lot of attention has been placed on cancer. Greenberg (1984), Horner and Chirikos (1987) and Schorr et al. (1989) found similar cancer mortality rates in urban and rural areas. Urban blacks had higher cancer incidence rates than rural blacks (Greenberg, Stevens, & Whitaker, 1985), however. Liff, Chow, and Greenberg (1991) found rural residents were diagnosed at later stages of cancer compared to urban residents.

No differences were found in mortality rates between urban and rural areas for pulmonary disease, diabetes mellitus, and atherosclerosis (Schorr et al., 1989). Rural Mexican Americans had higher rates of diabetes than the general population (Hanis et al., 1983), however. Cardiovascular and cerebrovascular disease mortality rates were higher in rural areas (Schorr et al., 1989). Barton, Combs, Miller, Hughes, and Cutter (1987) found gender differences in rates of hypertension in rural and urban areas. Moreover, race was a factor in rural cardiovascular mortality (Keil et al., 1985). Edwards, Parker, Burks, West, and Adams (1991) found higher cardiovascular risk factors for rural women than for urban women. Barger and Oldaker (1991) did not find a relationship between stress and lifestyle risk factors for cardiovascular disease. The high rate of risks in general for rural populations was of concern, however.

Miller, Stokes, and Clifford (1987) attributed discrepancies in mortality rates to differences in demographic structures in rural and urban areas; rural areas have a greater proportion of older adults. Wright, Champagne, Dever, and Clark (1985) controlled for age and race, and still found higher mortality rates in rural areas compared to urban areas. Similar results were found whether rural was defined as county population or metropolitan status. Contrary to the findings of Wright et al. (1985, 1993), in two separate studies, age-adjusted death rates differed little between urban and rural areas (Clifford & Brannon, 1985; Farmer, Stokes, Fiser, & Papini, 1991).

Substance Use.   The alcohol and drug consumption of rural populations has received considerable attention. Almost 60% of a sample of rural sixth and seventh graders reported using alcohol (Long & Boik, 1993). Children with poor self-concept and negative school attitudes in third and fourth grade were most likely to use alcohol in sixth and seventh grade. Higher rates of alcohol use were found for rural adolescents than for the rest of the nation (Sarvela & McClendon, 1987). Alcohol use in rural adolescents was significantly correlated to cigarette smoking (Sarvela & McClendon, 1983). Alcohol use decreased with age in older adults residing in rural areas (Christopherson, Escher, & Baunton, 1984).

Drug use may be higher in Mexican-American rural adolescents than white adolescents (Cockerham & Alster, 1983). Winfree and Griffiths (1983) found significantly less use of marijuana among rural adolescents and a trend toward conservatism in their attitudes about drugs. Social environmental factors were associated with drug use in rural adolescents in several studies (Goe, Napier,

& Bachtel, 1985; Napier, Goe, & Bachtel, 1984; Winfree & Griffiths, 1983). Drug-using rural and urban women in the Southeast did not differ in their crack use, sexual practices, and potential for HIV infection and transmission (Forney, Inciardi, & Lockwood, 1992).

   Mental Illness.   Wagenfeld (1990) reviewed research on the prevalence of mental disorders and concluded that further research is needed to determine the extent of mental illnesses in rural areas. Rates of depression in older rural adults have been found to be low (O'Hara, Kohourt, & Wallace, 1985). Hendricks and Turner (1988) found no differences between rural and urban elderly in rates of mental illness. Age, health and income had greater effects on depression than rurality. Blazer et al. (1985) found higher rates of major depressive disorders in an urban area as compared to a rural area. In a national study, no differences were found in depression scores between urban and rural older adults; however, the social network structures that predicted depression differed (Johnson et al., 1988). Depression in metropolitan elderly was found to be associated with intimate social relations, whereas in nonmetropolitan elderly, secondary social attachments were related to depression. Gender and education along with past depression scores predicted current depression scores in rural elderly (Wallace & O'Hara, 1992). Chronic medical problems, personal coping resources, and social support predicted depression in rural older adults (Linn & Husaini, 1985). Relocation also may be a factor in depressive symptoms of older adults (Colsher & Wallace, 1990).

   Farm wives did not differ in incidence of depressive symptoms although farm husbands had more depressive symptoms than nonfarm husbands (Lorenz, Conger, Montague, & Wickrama, 1993). Financial instability and stress were primary factors in depression for farmers (Belyea & Lobac, 1990). Perceived economic hardship and personal control mediated the relationship between financial stress and depression (Armstrong & Schulman, 1990). Support from spouses also buffered the relationship between stress and depression (Lorenz et al., 1993).

   Depression has been the focus of most articles on mental illness in rural areas. Few other mental health problems have been investigated. The etiology of suicide may differ between rural areas and urban areas (Lester, 1991). Abuse of mentally ill rural residents has been found; however, no comparison data with urban incidence was collected (Weiler & Buckwalter, 1992).

HEALTH NEEDS

Rural residents have been viewed as having greater health needs than urban residents due to inadequate resources and poorer health. Omishakin (1983) found that black farm workers needed improved health care and more information about environmental hazards. Rural residents experiencing cancer identified needs related to coping, support, information, interpersonal relations, reactions to cancer diagnosis, depression, and fear (Sullivan, Weinert, & Fulton, 1993). A study of rural care providers for those with cancer indicated that 66% had spiritual needs and 56% had emotional needs (Weinert & Bender, 1993). Moreover, rural health care providers identified many service needs for individuals with cancer, including personal and respite care (Burman, Steffes, & Weinert, 1994).

Slater and Black (1986) compared service needs of developmentally disabled residents in both rural and urban areas. The greatest needs were for medical/dental care, training, advocacy, counseling, sheltered apartments, and employment opportunities. Rural residents had been receiving services for a shorter period of time and were participating in fewer recreational, counseling, and sheltered employment activities than urban residents (Slater & Black, 1986). Disabled individuals identified health needs related to physical/emotional problems, completion of house and yard work, employment, and mobility (Omohundro, Schneider, Marr, & Grannenmann, 1983).

Rural elders identified needs for screening, health education, new health care therapies, and life management counseling (Davis et al., 1991). Franck (1979) found more similarities than differences between health needs of rural and urban older adults. For both urban and rural elderly, however, a variety of unmet needs existed. In a study of elderly at the time of discharge from the hospital, Schultz (1990) found that rural residents reported more skilled care needs than the urban elderly. Her work brings into question some of the earlier findings related to the role of the rural family in assisting the elderly. Leinbach (1988) reported statistically significant differences in needs for rural and urban elderly in several surveys. He argued that practical significance (as opposed to statistical significance) is limited because of very small differences in reported needs,

Health care provider perceptions often have been used to identify health needs. Roberto, Richter, Bottenberg, and MacCormack (1992) argued that this may be inappropriate for identifying the needs of rural elderly. Significant differences in perceived health problems were found between health care providers and rural elderly residents.

Critique

Consistently, rural dwellers have defined health functionally. Lack of urban comparison groups makes it difficult to draw valid conclusions, however. Whether a greater proportion of rural residents define health as the ability to work as compared to urban dwellers is not known. Moreover, the investigations of health beliefs of rural dwellers have focused on geographically distinct populations.

Physical and mental well-being of adults and older adults has received considerable attention, whereas the well-being of rural children and adolescents has been neglected. Although the typical profile of rural dwellers is one of poorer health, higher rates of acute and chronic illnesses, and greater health needs, few consistent differences were found in the research reviewed. Lack of consistency of findings is of concern and could be a result of several factors. First, certain aspects of rural living may predispose people to specific health problems, for example, the economic crises in farming lead to increased stress in farm families, and so higher rates of health problems would be anticipated. The same can be said for health needs. Some rural areas suffer from a lack of health care resources leading to greater unmet needs. The differences in health status and needs would not necessarily be consistent throughout all rural areas, however. Second, other demographic variables, such as race, socioeconomic status, and gender, may help explain some of the inconsistencies. For example, rural Mexican Americans had higher rates of diabetes than the general population (Hanis et al., 1983). Finally, methodological problems cannot be ignored. The examination of health, as well as health needs, has been fragmented by small samples, distinct and geographically separated groups, disparate definitions of health and health needs, and inconsistent measurement of degree of rurality. Consequently, it is difficult to draw valid conclusions about rural and urban health.

HEALTH-SEEKING BEHAVIOR

Health-seeking represents the range of activities that individuals undertake to promote or restore health, including health promotion/protective activities, self-management of health problems, use of informal resources such as the family network, and use of formal professional resources. Life styles, health beliefs, and resource availability affect health perception and health-related behaviors (Long & Weinert, 1992). For example, health-seeking behaviors of rural dwellers are strongly affected by reliance on informal networks of family and friends for the diagnosis and treatment of illness, and a distrust of "outsiders" and "newcomers" (Stein, 1987; Weinert & Long, 1987).

Health Promotion

Sexual Behavior. Older rural adolescents were more likely to have used contraception than younger adolescents (Scott, 1991). Religiosity was not related to abstinence from sexual intercourse in rural adolescents and contraceptive use was sporadic (McCormick, Izzo, & Folcik, 1985).

Dietary Habits. Steele and Spurgeon (1983) found dietary deficiencies in rural and urban black girls. Rural black children had an excess of caloric intake (Steele & Gallagher, 1985). Transition farm families with women employed off the farm or headed by widowed women had the poorest diets as opposed to traditional farm families who had the best nutrition (Hertzler, Caldwell, & Mark-Teo, 1987). Dietary habits of farmers may put them at risk for other problems because of exposure to harmful chemicals. People who ate more homegrown products had greater exposure to pesticides (Stehr-Green, Farrar, Burse, Royce, & Wohlleb, 1988). Older rural black women performed a variety of health-protective behaviors as well as harmful behaviors and the most common health-protective behavior was eating nutritionally sound diets (Wilson-Ford, 1992).

Protective Behaviors.   Using data from the 1985 National Interview Survey, Duelberg (1992) found racial differences in preventive health behavior of women. Rural/urban residency was found to modify the effect of race on health behavior. For example, no differences were found between urban and rural white women in their likelihood of obtaining a Pap test. Urban black women were more likely to have had a Pap test than rural black women, however. Rural women were more likely to use seat belts and urban women were more likely to have been smokers (Mansfield, Preston, & Crawford, 1989). Rural women who perceived more benefits from breast self-examination (BSE), fewer barriers to practicing BSE, and greater motivation were more likely to practice BSE (Gray, 1990). Rural parents who buckled up their children from birth were most likely to be currently using child restraints (Moss & Robin, 1988). Rural children had lower seatbelt use overall than urban children, however (Levey, Curry, & Levey, 1988).

Older Adults.   In older adults, perceptions of health were related to performance of preventive behaviors such as exercise (Lassey, Lassey, Carlson, & Sargent, 1985). Rural elders reported exercising and following a balanced diet in order to maintain their health (Davis et al., 1991). Johnson (1991) found that positive health practices related to nutrition, sleep, exercise, safe driving, and use of alcohol were practiced infrequently and inconsistently by rural residents, however. Social support was positively associated with health-promoting behaviors, but not to self-reported health status, for a group of rural elderly (Riffle, Yoho, & Sams, 1989).

Self-Management

In addition to health-promotion behaviors, a component of health-seeking is self-management of symptoms to restore health. Self-reliance and self-help were significant strategies used to cope with illness by rural persons (Weinert & Long, 1987). Formal resources were used only when self-management or lay resources failed to alleviate the symptoms or when the symptoms intensified (Mesaros, Malone, & Buehler, 1990). The time-line for rural women may be as long as 14 days from the time of symptom recognition to professional contact. This time-line is shortened for illness of a child, however. Self-reliance may lead to failure to seek appropriate help or failure to use the health services after seeking them out, with serious health consequences. Scharff (1987) found that rural dwellers often delayed seeking health care until they were gravely ill or incapacitated. This delay in seeking health care is consistent with their function-based definition of health (Lee, 1989; Ross, 1982; Weinert & Long, 1987).

Compliance.   Using unstructured interviews with rural African Americans, Roberson (1992) found only partial adherence with medical treatments. Treatments that are manageable, livable, and effective were sought by these rural residents. Although health care providers would classify these participants as "noncompliant," the rural African Americans saw themselves as doing a good job of managing their illnesses. Irvine (1989) and Roberson (1992) examined the health behaviors of rural residents with chronic illness. Less than one-fifth of diabetics questioned stayed on their diet every day; in addition, foot care and exercise were inadequately practiced (Irvine, 1989). Older rural adults identified a variety of barriers to management of hypertension including diet and weight problems, medication taking and side-effects, fears regarding potential strokes, decreased motivation, and lack of support from significant others (Whetstone & Reid, 1991).

Informal Social Support

Although the role of social support in health has been recognized and studied since the 1970s, the concept has been known for eons in the guise of friendship, community cohesion, caring, or unconditional positive regard (Tilden, 1985). Rural pregnant women had less affirmation support, smaller network size, longer duration of relationships, greater frequency of contact, and a greater sense of loss of social support than a comparable group of pregnant urban women (Pass, 1991). Perceptions of social support varied dramatically for urban and rural dwellers based on health status, caregiving status, and living arrangements (Burman & Weinert, 1994). Rural men whose wives had multiple sclerosis (MS) reported less overall social support, fewer social network resources, less support from neighbors, and less involvement with or reliance on religion (Weinert & Long, 1993). Weinert and Long concluded that men living with chronically ill spouses in rural areas were at considerable risk for stress, fatigue, and the development of physical and psychosocial illnesses.

Family/Kin Support.   Crawford and Preston (1991) found that the family was an especially important source of support for rural residents and women in maintaining selected health promotion activities. Magilvy, Congdon, and Martinez (1993) described "circles of informal care" of both healthy and frail older rural adults, which included family, friends, and neighbors who provided assistance with meals, household tasks, shopping, personal care, health-related care, errands, transportation, and companionship. Powers and Kivett (1992) reported that both expected and actual levels of assistance from kin declined as the level of consanguineous kin and associated affinal ties decreased. The level of support by kin groups was mainly a function of geographic distance to kin and the norms of obligation. Amato (1993) found, based on a large national probability sample, that for urbanites as well as small-town dwellers, the further away family members lived, the less likely they were to be mentioned as sources of assistance and the more likely the respondents were to mention friends.

The elderly living in rural areas did not have especially strong family ties as measured by the frequency of contact with their children (Krout, 1988). Impaired rural elderly were less likely to live with a child than were impaired elderly living in larger cities (Lee, Dwyer, & Coward, 1990). These findings have serious implications as the lack of health and other services in rural areas is not counterbalanced by any greater availability of an adult offspring to provide informal assistance to their aging rural parents. Informal caregiving is an essential component of in-home care for community elders in rural areas (Newhouse & McAuley, 1988). Rural dwellers who had cared for a loved one with cancer indicated that the strain of caregiving was increased due to the limited formal resources, especially for those living in the frontier areas (Buehler & Lee, 1992).

Community Support.   The rural setting is often considered to be an environment with informal supportive resources, which can enable individuals to manage health and illness. A hallmark of rural communities is the ability and willingness to enter into joint activities at times such as harvesting and branding or to help in individual and family crises (Weinert & Long, 1991). Rural families placed special importance on neighbors as sources of informal help and support and were relied on for support in dealing with health problems much more often than formal agencies or professional care providers (Long & Weinert, 1989; Weinert & Long, 1987, 1990). Some families who lost their family farms felt that they had lost some or all of their neighbors as well (Graham, 1986).

Van Nostrand (1993) noted the commonly held belief that the nonmetropolitan elderly benefit from a closely knit community, have a better social support network, and are more involved in religious activities. Yet, he reported that there is little evidence that rural elderly have a more closely knit community although their social support networks may be a little larger.

Professional Resources

Rural elderly tended not to consult health care providers before using over-the-counter drugs or when experiencing side effects from prescription drugs

(Johnson, 1988). In another study, the elderly managed most symptoms them-selves, sought consultation from family members or friends, and tended not to seek help from the formal care system (Stoller & Forster, 1992). Informal sup-ports compensated for lack of formal health care when illness struck (Scott & Roberto, 1988) and farm couples showed a reluctance to use outsiders and relied heavily on spouse, family, and friends (Cook & Tyler, 1989). Windley and Scheidt (1983), in a study of psychologically vulnerable rural elderly, found that utilization of basic community services is a necessary part of independent living and that the informal helping network assisted the more vulnerable elderly in obtaining these services. Contrary to prevailing stereotypes, rural chroni-cally ill were not collectively isolated from service contact; service utilization was affected by a variety of factors including client age, maladaptive behav-iors, and geographic location (Sommers, 1989).

In a study with 200 urban and rural residents, stigma in rural areas was a much stronger deterrent to seeking mental health care than in urban areas (Rost et al., 1993). Moreover, rural residents preferred to use primary caregivers ex-cept for serious mental illness (Flaskerud & Kviz, 1982). Some rural residents described a sense of powerlessness in their interactions with the health care system (Counts & Boyle, 1987).

Levey et al. (1988) found that rural children, irrespective of income, had less access to pediatric care, greater travel time to providers, discontinuity of well care and sick care, lower seat belt use, less likelihood of well visits, and less attentiveness by providers to behavioral and developmental issues than urban children. In the case of young children, use of services is dependent on parents' beliefs about well-child care, their concept of illness, and their notion of when care is required (Crawford & Preston, 1991).

A review of the research published in the 1980s indicated that rural elderly were relatively disadvantaged in terms of both health status and access to health care services and had little advantage over the urban elderly in their access to informal sources of care (Dwyer, Lee, & Coward, 1990). Coward, Cutler, and Mullens (1990) reported that it was primarily the impaired elderly in large cit-ies who experienced a lack of informal assistance. Consistent with this finding is the notion that in small towns, where social networks are geographically clustered more closely, the elderly may find it easier to keep in touch (Amato, 1993).

Health Information

Preferences for acquisition of health-related information have been explored. Briley, Owens, Gilham, and Sharplin (1990) found little difference in sources of nutrition information between urban and rural elderly. Elderly preferred writ-ten materials as a source of health information (Briley et al., 1990; Connell & Crawford, 1988). Rural youth indicated that both the media and their teachers were important sources of drug and alcohol information (Sarvela, Newcomb, & Littlefield, 1988).

Critique

Health promotion research in rural populations is highly fragmented and such factors as race, gender, and age may be more critical than place of residence. The research is not conclusive due to the limited number of studies, lack of replication, demographic differences within the rural population, and the dearth of comparison studies of rural and urban samples. A critical factor in health-seeking is the characteristic of self-reliance, which may be associated with delay in seeking health care (Long & Weinert, 1989). Yet, it is difficult to evaluate the causal link between self-reliance and delay in health seeking or to determine if this characteristic is generalizable to other rural dwellers. Self-care practices and patterns of seeking help when self-care practices prove ineffective are discussed in the literature. Little substantive research has been conducted to validate these patterns or to compare them to those of urban residents, however.

The beneficial outcomes of appropriate and adequate social support are widely accepted. And the rural research literature focuses a fair amount of attention on the role of support and the sources of support, particularly from family, neighbors, and community. The work of Burman and Weinert (1994) and Weinert and Long (1993) indicated that factors such as chronic illness, caregiving status, and living arrangements may be just as influential as rural residence. Likewise, social support and social network patterns need to be carefully examined as they vary based on place of rural residence such as a small town in contrast to an isolated farm or ranch. Virtually no research was located that looked at the role of support for special rural populations such as the reservation Native American.

Care must be taken to avoid overgeneralization about the health behaviors of rural individuals. Miller, Stokes, and Clifford (1987) noted that there are many rural populations made up of different race, gender, ethnic, and age groups, and that ultimately each community will generate its own pattern of health and illness. Cutler and Coward's (1988) work demonstrated the heterogeneity of rural environments and emphasized the inadequacy of simple residential dichotomies. Clearly, the future research on rural health-seeking must take these admonitions into careful consideration.

SUMMARY AND FUTURE RESEARCH DIRECTIONS

Interest in rural health and rural nursing has grown dramatically in the past 10 years. Yet, health and health-seeking have not been adequately examined.

Overall, the body of rural research and rural nursing research is severely limited. Even with the addition of research from all related disciplines, the knowledge base is seriously fragmented. Consequently, limited research is available to guide the practice of rural nursing.

One effort to develop a rural nursing theory has used both qualitative and quantitative methods to learn about the culture and health of rural dwellers in a sparsely populated state (Long & Weinert, 1989; Weinert & Long, 1987, 1990, 1991). Key rural concepts have been identified: work and health beliefs, isolation and distance, independence and self-reliance, lack of anonymity, outsider/insider, and oldtimer/newcomer. Initial relational statements have been developed and are being tested. First, rural dwellers define health primarily as the ability to work, to be productive, and to do usual tasks. Second, rural dwellers are self-reliant and resist accepting help from those viewed as outsiders. Help, including health care, is usually sought through an informal rather than a formal system. Third, health care providers in rural areas must deal with a lack of anonymity and much greater role diffusion than providers in urban or suburban settings.

Although this emerging theory provides exciting potential for the development of a sound knowledge base, limited evaluation of the tenets of the theory has been done. Replication with the other groups in sparsely populated states, empirical testing of the relational statements, and exploration of the key concepts with a variety of rural populations is needed. Further definition of common and locale-specific conditions and characteristics of rural populations also is needed.

Rural studies suffer from the age-old problems of small sample size, lack of random sampling, and cross-sectional designs. Those studies that were conducted using large existing data bases often were constrained by limitations of appropriate questions and the delineation of rurality.

In addition to these common design problems, rural research has been constrained by unique flaws. Operationalization and measurement of rurality was a serious problem in the research reviewed. There was little consistency of measurement across studies, and in some studies no definition of rural was provided. Care should be taken when reporting and reading rural research so that the myth that rural is rural is rural is not perpetuated. The relative measure of rurality (miles to emergency room and the population of the county) proposed by Weinert and Boik (1993) may prove to be a fruitful approach for rural nursing research, but testing across populations must be done.

Many studies were limited to a given population, such as those dwelling in a particular state, with no replication or testing with other populations. Conversely, researchers must guard against specific groups living in rural areas being swept up into generalizations about rural dwellers. For example, although Native Americans live in rural America, many of their health problems are more like those of other oppressed peoples in inner cities rather than their rural counterparts.

Moreover, targeted research programs did not exist to any great degree, particularly within nursing. Very few studies were focused on the same topic area and lacked the in-depth investigation and knowledge development characteristic of programs of research. In addition, certain critical rural health issues, such as relocation for either temporary or long-term health care, received little attention.

To address the limitations in the research a variety of approaches should be considered. Multi-site, cluster, and collaborative studies would lead to a deeper understanding of rural concepts. Collaboration, within nursing and across disciplines and institutions, is imperative in rural research because those best suited for conducting rural research often are located in low resource institutions.

Well-designed studies using carefully conceptualized definitions of rurality need to be conducted to delineate rural/urban differences while accounting for the effects of other demographic variables such as race and socioeconomic status. Geographic isolation, inaccessible and unavailable health care resources, cultural antagonism, and economic hardships have been identified as central issues in rural health. More extensive study is needed within rural populations and between rural and urban populations using concepts relevant to these issues. Evaluation, adaptation, or development of measurement instruments that are valid, reliable, and sensitive to rural populations are critical. The work by Goeppinger, Doyle, Charlton, and Lorig (1988) is an example of this type of psychometric evaluation.

Innovative methods to capture adequately the picture of rural life and rural health needs should be considered. Magilvy, Congdon, Nelson, and Craig (1992) used photography as a method imbedded in an ethnographic investigation of home care of rural older adults and reported that it fostered data generation, elicited participants' stories, and illustrated patterns of rural aging. Expanding communication technologies are especially suited to rural areas, allowing electronic linkages between geographically distant individuals and health care providers. Such technologies could be used in intervention research, for example, to facilitate support between chronically ill rural residents or to teach and evaluate health promotion strategies.

The claim often made is that nursing research as a discipline is in its adolescence. Rural nursing research has not achieved even that level of development. Recently interest in rural health issues has increased dramatically and is reflected in federal research initiatives. Nursing is amassing the critical cadre of researchers with interest in rural issues and who possess the appropriate research skills and background. The priority for researchers is the development of rural nursing theory and an empirically substantiated knowledge base relevant to health and health care needs of rural populations. A knowledge base to guide rural nursing practice is an achievable and essential goal for nursing science. Nursing is capable of responding to "the challenge to expand and adapt health resources so that the myths surrounding rural health and well-being can more closely approximate the rural reality" (Weinert & Long, 1990, p. 71).

REFERENCES

Adams, T., & Perkin, J. (1985). The prevalence of intestinal parasites in children living in an unincorporated area in rural northern Florida. *Journal of School Health, 55,* 76–78.

Amato, P. (1993). Urban-rural differences in helping friends and family members. *Social Psychology Quarterly, 56,* 249–262.

Amato, P., & Zuo, J. (1992). Rural poverty, urban poverty, and psychological well-being. *The Sociological Quarterly, 33,* 229–240.

Armstrong, P., & Schulman, M. (1990). Financial strain and depression among farm operators: The role of perceived economic hardship and personal control. *Rural Sociology, 55,* 475–493.

Baker, S., & Kotelchuck, M. (1989). Birthweight-specific mortality: Important inequalities remain. *The Journal of Rural Health, 5,* 155–170.

Barger, S., & Oldaker, S. (1991). A determination of stress and risk factors for cardiovascular disease in a rural population. In A. Bushy (Ed.), *Rural Nursing* (Vol. 1, pp. 229–242). Newbury Park, CA: Sage.

Barton, S., Coombs, D., Miller, H., Hughes, G., & Cutter, G. (1987). Comparison of hypertension prevalence and control in 5237 rural and urban Alabama residents. *Southern Medical Journal, 80,* 1220–1223.

Belshe, R., Van Voris, L., & Mufson, M. (1983). Impact of viral respiratory diseases on infants and young children in a rural and urban area of southern West Virginia. *American Journal of Epidemiology, 117,* 467–474.

Belyea, M., & Lobao, L. (1990). Psychosocial consequences of agricultural transformation: The farm crisis and depression. *Rural Sociology, 55,* 58–75.

Berkowitz, A., & Perkins, H. (1984). Stress among farm women: Work and family as interacting systems. *Journal of Marriage and the Family, 46,* 161–166.

Bigbee, J. (1987). Stressful life events among women: A rural-urban comparison. *The Journal of Rural Health, 3,* 39–51.

Bigbee, J. (1988). Rurality, stress, and illness among women: A pilot study. *Health Care for Women International, 9,* 43–61.

Bigbee, J. (1990). Stressful life events and illness occurrence in rural versus urban women. *Journal of Community Health Nursing, 7,* 105–113.

Bigbee, J. (1991). The concept of hardiness as applied to rural nursing. In A. Bushy (Ed.), *Rural Nursing* (Vol. 1, pp. 39–58). Newbury Park, CA: Sage.

Blazer, D., George, L., Landerman, R., Pennybacker, M., Melville, M., Woodbury, M., Manton, K., Jordon, K., & Locke, B. (1985). Psychiatric disorders. A rural/urban comparison. *Archives of General Psychiatry, 42,* 651–656.

Briley, M., Owens, M., Gilham, M., & Sharplin, S. (1990). Sources of nutrition information for rural and urban elderly adults. *Journal of the American Dietetic Association, 90,* 986–987.

Brown, K. (1990). Connected independence: A paradox of rural health. *Journal of Rural Community Psychology, 11,* 51–64.

Buehler, J., & Lee, H. (1992). Exploration of home care resources for rural families with cancer. *Cancer Nursing, 15,* 299–308.

Burman, M., Steffes, M., & Weinert, C. (1994). Cancer home care in Montana. *Home Health Care Services Quarterly, 4,* 37–52.

Burman, M., & Weinert, C. (1994). *Social support and networks in rural and urban America.* Unpublished manuscript. Montana State University, College of Nursing, Bozeman, MT.

Calonge, B., Petersen, L., Miller, R., & Marshall, G. (1993). Human immunodeficiency virus seroprevalence in primary care practices in the United States. *Western Journal of Medicine, 158,* 148–152.

Christopherson, V., Escher, M., & Baunton, B. (1984). Reasons for drinking among the elderly in rural Arizona. *Journal of Studies on Alcohol, 45,* 417–423.

Clifford, W., & Brannon, Y. (1985). Rural-urban differentials in mortality. *Rural Sociology, 50,* 210–224.

Cockerham, W., & Alster, J. (1983). A comparison of marijuana use among Mexican-American and Anglo rural youth utilizing a matched-set analysis. *The International Journal of the Addictions, 18,* 759–767.

Colsher, P., & Wallace, R. (1990). Health and social antecedents of relocation in rural elderly persons. *Journal of Gerontology, 45,* S32–S38.

Connell, C., & Crawford, C. (1988). How people obtain their health information. *Public Health Reports, 103,* 189–195.

Cook, J., & Tyler, J. (1989). Help-seeking attitudes of North Dakota farm couples. *Journal of Rural Community Psychology, 10,* 17–28.

Cordes, S. (1985). Biopsychosocial imperative from the rural perspective. *Social Science in Medicine, ?1,* 1373–1379.

Cordes, S. (1989). The changing rural environment and the relationship to health services and rural development. *Health Services Research, 23,* 57–78.

Counts, M., & Boyle, J. (1987). Nursing, health, and policy within a community context. *Advances in Nursing Science, 9*(3), 12–23.

Coward, R., & Cutler, S. (1988). The concept of a continuum of residence: Comparing activities of daily living among the elderly. *Journal of Rural Studies, 4,* 159–168.

Coward, R., Cutler, S., & Mullens, R. (1990). Residential differences in the composition of the helping networks of impaired elders. *Family Relations, 39,* 44–50.

Crawford, C., & Preston, D. (1991). Differences in specific sources of social support for four healthy behaviors. In A. Bushy (Ed.), *Rural Nursing* (Vol. 1, pp 215–227). Newbury Park, CA: Sage.

Crowder, M., Higgins, H., & Frost, J. (1987). Rubella susceptibility in young women of rural east Texas: 1980 and 1985. *Texas Medicine, 83,* 43–47.

Cutler, S., & Coward, R. (1988). Residence differences in the health status of elders. *Journal of Rural Health, 4,* 11–26.

Davis, D., Henderson, M., Boothe, A., Douglass, M., Faria, S., Kennedy, D., Kitchens, E., & Weaver, M. (1991). An interactive perspective on the health beliefs and practices of rural elders. *Journal of Gerontological Nursing, 17*(5), 11–16.

Duelberg, S. (1992). Preventive health behavior among black and white women in urban and rural areas. *Social Science and Medicine, 34,* 191–198.

Duncan, S., Volk, R., & Lewis, R. (1988). The influence of financial stressors upon farm husbands and wives' well-being and family life satisfaction. In R. Marotz-Baden, C. B. Hennon, & T. Brubaker (Eds.), *Family in rural America: Stress, adaptation and revitalization* (pp. 32–39). St. Paul, MN: National Council of Family Relations.

Dunkin, J., Holzwarth, C., & Stratton, T. (1993). Assessment of rural family hardiness: A foundation for intervention. In S. L. Feetham, S. Meister, J. Bell, & C. Gillis (Eds.), *The nursing of families* (pp. 247–255). Newbury Park, CA: Sage.

Dwyer, J., Lee, G., & Coward, R. (1990). The health status, health services utilization, and support networks of the rural elderly: A decade review. *The Journal of Rural Health, 6,* 379–398.

Dwyer, J., & Miller, M. (1990). Determinants of primary caregiver stress and burden: Area of residence and the caregiving networks of frail elders. *The Journal of Rural Health, 6,* 161–184.

Edwards, K., Parker, D., Burks, C., West, A., & Adams, M. (1991). Cardiovascular risk: Among black and white rural-urban low income women. *The Association of Black Nursing Faculty Journal, 2,* 72–76.

Eggebeen, D., & Lichter, D. (1993). Health and well-being among rural Americans: Variations across the life course. *The Journal of Rural Health, 9,* 86–98.

Farmer, F., Stokes, C., Fiser, R., & Papini, D. (1991). Poverty, primary care and age-specific mortality. *Journal of Rural Health, 7,* 153–169.

Flaskerud, J., & Kviz, F. (1982). Resources rural consumers indicate they would use for mental health problems. *Community Mental Health Journal, 18,* 107–119.

Flaskerud, J., & Kviz, F. (1983). Rural attitudes toward and knowledge of mental illness and treatment resources. *Hospital and Community Psychiatry, 34,* 229–233.

Forney, M., Inciardi, J., & Lockwood, D. (1992). Exchanging sex for crack-cocaine: A comparison of women from rural and urban communities. *Journal of Community Health, 17*(2), 73–85.

Franck, P. (1979). A survey of health needs of older adults in Northwest Johnson County, Iowa. *Nursing Research, 28,* 360–364.

Geller, J., Bultena, G., & Lasley, P. (1988). Stress on the farm: A test of the life-events perspective among Iowa farm operators. *Journal of Rural Health, 4,* 43–57.

Geller, J., Ludtke, R., & Stratton, T. (1990). Nonfatal farm injuries in North Dakota: A sociological analysis. *Journal of Rural Health, 6,* 185–196.

Goe, W., Napier, T., & Bachtel, D. (1985). Use of marijuana among rural high school students: A test of a facilitative-constraint model. *Rural Sociology, 50,* 409–426.

Goeppinger, J., Doyle, M., Charlton, S., & Lorig, K. (1988). A nursing perspective on the assessment of function in persons with arthritis. *Journal of Nursing and Health, 11,* 321–331.

Gold, M., & Franks, P. (1989). Farming: Primary prevention for hypertension? Effects of employment type on blood pressure. *Journal of Rural Health, 5,* 257–265.

Graham, K. (1986). *A Description of the transition experiences of 28 New York State farm families forced from their farms: 1982–1986.* Unpublished master's thesis. Cornell University, Ithaca, NY.

Gray, M. (1990). Factors related to practice of breast self-examination in rural women. *Cancer Nursing, 13,* 100–107.

Greenberg, M. (1984). Changing cancer mortality patterns in the rural United States. *Rural Sociology, 49,* 145–153.

Greenberg, M., Stevens, J., & Whitaker, J. (1985). Cancer incidence rates among blacks in urban and rural Georgia, 1978–1982. *American Journal of Public Health, 75,* 683–684.

Gross, T., Silverman, P. R., Bloch, A., Smith, T., & Rogers, G. (1989). An outbreak of tuberculosis in rural Delaware. *American Journal of Epidemiology, 129,* 362–371.

Halpert, B., & Zimmerman, M. (1986). The health status of the 'old-old': A reconsideration. *Social Science and Medicine, 22,* 893–899.

Hanis, C., Ferrell, R., Barton, S., Aguilar, L., Garza-Ibarra, A., Tulloch, B., Garcia, C., & Schull, W. (1983). Diabetes among Mexican Americans in Starr County, Texas. *American Journal of Epidemiology, 118,* 659–672.

Hassinger, E. (1982). *Rural health organizations.* Ames, IA: Iowa State University Press.

Heffernan, W., & Heffernan, J. (1986). Impact of the farm crisis on rural families and communities. *Rural Sociology, 6,* 160–170.

Hendricks, J., & Turner, H. (1988). Social dimensions of mental illness among rural elderly populations. *International Journal of Aging and Human Development, 26,* 169–190.

Hertzler, A., Caldwell, J., & Mark-Teo, M. (1987). Factors related to dietary status of limited resource farm families: A case study. *Journal of Rural Health, 3,* 47–60.

Hewitt, M. (1992). Defining rural areas: Impact on health care policy and research. In W. Gesler & T. Ricketts (Eds.), *Health in rural North America* (pp. 25–54). New Brunswick: Rutgers University Press.

Horner, R., & Chirikos, T. (1987). Survivorship differences in geographical comparisons of cancer mortality: An urban-rural analysis. *International Journal of Epidemiology, 16,* 184–189.

Hunt, R., Beck, J., Lemke, J., Kohout, F., & Wallace, R. (1985). Edentulism and oral health problems among elderly rural Iowans: The Iowa 65+ rural health study. *American Journal of Public Health, 75,* 1177–1181.

Ide, B. (1992/4th quarter). A process model of rural nursing. *The Texas Journal of Rural Health,* 30–34.

Ide, B., & Arquistain, M. (1993, September). *Development and testing of a farm/ranch stress scale.* Paper presented at the Conference on Instrumentation in Nursing, Tucson, AR.

Irvine, A. (1989). Self care behaviors in a rural population with diabetes. *Patient Education and Counseling, 18,* 3–13.

Johnson, J. (1988). The drug-taking practices of the rural elderly. *Applied Nursing Research, 1,* 128–131.

Johnson, J. (1991). Health-care practices of the rural aged. *Journal of Gerontological Nursing, 17,* 15–19.

Johnson, T., Hendricks, J., Turner, H., Stallones, I., Marx, M., & Garrity, T. (1988). Social networks and depression among the elderly: Metropolitan/nonmetropolitan comparisons. *Journal of Rural Health, 4,* 72–83.

Jordan, S., & Hargrove, D. (1987). Implications of an empirical application of categorical definitions of rural. *Journal of Rural Community Psychology, 8,* 14–29.

Keil, J., Saunders, D., Lackland, D., Weinrich, M., Hudson, M., Gastright, J., Baroody, N., O'Bryan, E., & Zmyslinski, R. (1985). Acute myocardial infarction: Period prevalence, case fatality, and comparison of black and white cases in urban and rural areas of South Carolina. *American Health Journal, 109,* 776–784.

Kivett, V. (1985). Rural-urban differences in the physical and mental health of older adults. *Journal of Applied Gerontology, 4*(2), 9–19.

Krout, J. (1988). Rural versus urban differences in elderly parents' contact with their children, *Gerontologist, 28,* 198–203.

Krout, J. (1989). Rural versus urban differences in health dependence among the elderly population. *International Journal of Aging and Human Development, 28,* 141–156.

Lassey, M., Lassey, W., Carlson, J., & Sargent, M. (1985). Health maintenance antecedents among older citizens in rural and urban communities. *Journal of Rural Studies, 1*, 185–191.

Lavsky-Shulan, M., Wallace, R., Kohout, F., Lemke, J., Morris, M., & Smith, I. (1985). Prevalence and functional correlates of low back pain in the elderly: The Iowa 65+ rural health study. *Journal of American Geriatric Society, 33*, 23–28.

Lee, G., Dwyer, J., & Coward, R. (1990). Residential location and proximity to children among impaired elderly parents. *Rural Sociology, 55*, 579–589.

Lee, H. (1989). *Quantitative validation of health perceptions in rural persons.* Unpublished manuscript, Montana State University, College of Nursing, Bozeman, MT.

Lee, H. (1991a). Definitions of rural: A review of the literature. In A. Bushy (Ed.), *Rural nursing* (Vol. 1, pp. 7–20). Newbury Park, CA: Sage.

Lee, H. (1991b). Relationship of hardiness and current life events to perceived health in rural adults. *Research in Nursing & Health, 14*, 351–359.

Lee, H. (1993). Health perceptions of middle, "new middle," and older rural adults. *Family and Community Health, 16*, 19–27.

Leinbach, R. (1988). Differences in need among the rural and urban aged: Statistical versus practical significance. *Journal of Rural Health, 4*, 27–34.

Lester, D. (1991). The etiology of suicide and homicide in urban and rural America. *Journal of Rural Community Psychology, 12*, 15–27.

Levey, L., Curry, J., & Levey, S. (1988). Rural-urban differences in access to Iowa child health services. *Journal of Rural Health, 4*, 59–72.

Liff, J., Chow, W., & Greenberg, R. (1991). Rural-urban differences in stage at diagnosis. Possible relationship to cancer screening. *Cancer, 67*, 1454–1459.

Linn, J., & Husaini, B. (1985). Chronic medical problems, coping resources, and depression: A longitudinal study of rural Tennesseans. *American Journal of Community Psychology, 13*, 733–742.

Long, K. (1993). The concept of health: Rural perspectives. *The Nursing Clinics of North America, 28*, 123–130.

Long, K., & Boik, R. (1993). Predicting alcohol use in rural children: A longitudinal study. *Nursing Research, 42*, 79–86.

Long, K., & Weinert, C. (1989). Rural nursing: Developing the theory base. *Scholarly Inquiry in Nursing Practice, 3*, 113–127.

Long, K., & Weinert, C. (1992). Description and perceptions of health among rural and urban adults with multiple sclerosis. *Research in Nursing & Health, 15*, 335–342.

Lorenz, F., Conger, R., Montague, R., & Wickrama, K. (1993). Economic conditions, spouse support, and psychological distress of rural husbands and wives. *Rural Sociology, 58*, 247–268.

Magilvy, J., Congdon, J., Nelson, J., & Craig, C. (1992). Visions of rural aging: Use of photographic method in gerontological research. *The Gerontologist, 32*, 253–257.

Magilvy, J., Congdon, J., & Martinez, R. (1993). *Circles of care: Home care and community support for rural older adults.* Unpublished manuscript. University of Colorado Health Sciences Center, Denver, CO.

Mansfield, P., Preston, D., & Crawford, C. (1988). Rural-urban differences in women's psychological well-being. *Health Care for Women International, 9*, 289–304.

Mansfield, P., Preston, D., & Crawford, C. (1989). The health behaviors of rural women: Comparisons with an urban sample. *Health Values, 16*(6), 12–20.

Marotz-Baden, R. (1988). Stressors: A rural-urban comparison. In R. Marotz-Baden, C. B. Hennon, & T. H. Brubaker (Eds.), *Family in rural America: Stress, adaptation and revitalization* (pp. 74–82). St. Paul, MN: National Council of Family Relations.

McCormick, N., Izzo, A., & Folcik, J. (1985). Adolescents' values, sexuality, and contraception in a rural New York county. *Adolescence, 20*, 385–395.

McCulloch, B. (1991). Health and health maintenance profiles of older rural women, 1976–1986. In A. Bushy (Ed.), *Rural Nursing* (Vol. 1, pp. 281–298). Newbury Park, CA: Sage.

McGhee, J. (1984). The influence of qualitative assessments of the social and physical environment on the morale of the rural elderly. *American Journal of Community Psychology, 12*, 709–722.

McManus, M., Newacheck, P., & Weader, R. (1990). Metropolitan and nonmetropolitan adolescents: Differences in demographic and health characteristics. *Journal of Rural Health, 6*, 39–51.

Mesaros, J., Malone, M., & Buehler, J. (1990). *Symptom-action time line process: Patterns of responses to symptoms in rural residents.* Unpublished manuscript. Montana State University, College of Nursing, Bozeman, MT.

Miller, M., Stokes, C., & Clifford, W. (1987). A comparison of the rural-urban mortality differential for deaths from all causes, cardiovascular disease and cancer. *Journal of Rural Health, 3*, 23–34.

Miller, W., Qualtere-Burcher, P., Labuer, C., Rockow, J., & Bauman, K. (1990). AIDS knowledge and attitudes among adolescents in the rural Southwest. *Journal of Rural Health, 6*, 246–255.

Mookherjee, H. (1992). Perceptions of well-being by metropolitan and nonmetropolitan populations in the United States. *Journal of Social Psychology, 132*, 513–524.

Moss, J., & Robin, S. (1988). The relationship of parental perceptions and experiences to car seat use in rural children. *Journal of Pediatric Nursing, 3*, 103–109.

Napier, T., Goe, R., & Bachtel, D. (1984). An assessment of the influence of peer association and identification on drug use among rural high school students. *Journal of Drug Education, 14*, 227–247.

Newhouse, J., & McAuley, W. (1988). Use of informal in-home care of rural elders. In R. Marotz-Baden, C. B. Hennon, & T. Brubaker (Eds.), *Family in rural America: Stress, adaptation and revitalization* (pp. 233–239). St. Paul, MN: National Council of Family Relations.

Office of Management and Budget. (1983). Metropolitan statistical areas (NTIS No. PB83–218891). Washington, DC: Government Printing Office.

O'Hara, M., Kohout, F., & Wallace, R. (1985). Depression among the rural elderly. A study of prevalence and correlates. *The Journal of Nervous and Mental Disease, 173*, 582–589.

Omishakin, M. (1983). Assessment of health needs of black agricultural workers in mid-delta of Mississippi, USA. *Journal of the Royal Society of Health, 103*, 239–241.

Omohundro, J., Schneider, M., Marr, J., & Grannenmann, B. (1983). A four-county needs assessment of rural disabled people. *Journal of Rehabilitation, 49*(4), 19–24.

Pass, C. (1991). Social support and sex role orientation: A comparison of rural and urban pregnant women. In A. Bushy (Ed.), *Rural Nursing* (Vol. 1, pp 146–157). Newbury Park, CA: Sage.

Powers, E., & Kivett, V. (1992). Kin expectations and kin support among rural older adults. *Rural Sociology, 57*, 194–215.

Pratt, D. (1990). Occupational health and the rural worker: Agriculture, mining and logging. *Journal of Rural Health, 6,* 399–417.

Preston, D., & Crawford, C. (1990). A study of community differences in stress among the elderly: Implications for community health nursing. *Public Health Nursing, 7,* 229–235.

Preston, D., & Mansfield, P. (1984). An exploration of stressful life events, illness, and coping among the rural elderly. *The Gerontologist, 24,* 490–494.

Preston, D., & Mansfield, P. (1991). Assessing the health status of rural people: An analysis of American studies 1980–1985. *Advances in Health Education and Promotion, 3,* 243–296.

Quevillon, R., & Lee, H. (1983). Social involvement as a predictor of subjective well-being among the rural institutionalized aged. *International Journal of Behavioral Geriatrics, 1,* 13–19.

Riffle, K., Yoho, J., & Sams, J. (1989). Health-promoting behaviors, perceived social support, and self-reported health of Appalachian elderly. *Public Health Nursing, 6,* 204–211.

Roberson, M. (1992). The meaning of compliance: Patient perspectives. *Qualitative Health Research, 2,* 7–26.

Roberto, K., Richter, J., Bottenberg, D., & MacCormack, R. (1992). Provider/client views. Health-care needs of the rural elderly. *Journal of Gerontological Nursing, 18*(5), 31–37.

Robinson, D., & Comstock, G. (1992). Tuberculosis in a small semi-rural county. *Public Health Reports, 107,* 179–182.

Ross, H. (1982). Women and wellness: Defining, attaining, and maintaining health in Eastern Canada. *Dissertation Abstracts International, 42,* 5175A. (University Microfilms No. DA8212624)

Rost, K., Smith, G., & Taylor, J. (1993). Rural-urban differences in stigma and the use of care for depressive disorders. *Journal of Rural Health, 9,* 57–62.

Salmi, L., Weiss, H., Peterson, P., Spengler, R., Sattin, R., & Anderson, H. (1989). Fatal farm injuries among young children. *Pediatrics, 83,* 267–271.

Sarvela, P., & McClendon, E. (1987). Early adolescent alcohol abuse in rural Northern Michigan. *Community Mental Health Journal, 23,* 183–191.

Sarvela, P., & McClendon, E. (1983). Correlates of early adolescent peer and personal substance use in rural northern Michigan. *Journal of Youth and Adolescence, 12,* 319–332.

Sarvela, P., Newcomb, P., & Littlefield, E. (1988, June/July). Sources of drug and alcohol information among rural youth. *Health Education,* 27–31.

Scharff, J. (1987). *The nature and scope of rural nursing: Distinctive characteristics.* Unpublished master's thesis. Montana State University, Bozeman, MT.

Scheidt, R. (1984). A taxonomy of well-being for small-town elderly: A case for rural diversity. *The Gerontologist, 24,* 84–90.

Scheidt, R. (1986). Mental health of small-town Kansas elderly: A report from the Great Plains. *American Journal of Community Psychology, 14,* 541–554.

Schorr, V., Crabtree, D., Wagner, D., & Wetterau, P. (1989). Differences in rural and urban mortality: Implications for health education and promotion. *Journal of Rural Health, 5,* 67–80.

Schultz, A. (1990). Rural/urban differences in health care needs of the elderly after hospital discharge to home. *Dissertation Abstracts International, 52,* 5761B. (University Microfilms No. DA 9204799).

Scott, R. (1991). Attitudes, behaviors, and knowledge regarding contraceptive use among adolescents in Loudon County, Tennessee. In A. Bushy (Ed.), *Rural Nursing* (Vol. 1, pp. 173–186). Newbury, CA: Sage Publications.

Slater, M., & Black, P. (1986). Urban-rural differences in the delivery of community services: Wisconsin as a case in point. *Mental Retardation, 24,* 153–161.

Smith-Rooker, J., Garrett, A., Hodges, L., & Shue, V. (1992). Prevalence of Glioblastoma Multiform subjects with prior herbicide exposure. *Journal of Neuroscience Nursing, 24,* 260–264.

Sommers, I. (1989). Geographic location and mental health service utilization among the chronically mentally ill. *Community Mental Health Journal, 25,* 132–144.

Stallones, L. (1989). Fatal unintentional injuries among Kentucky farm children: 1979 to 1985. *Journal of Rural Health, 5,* 246–256.

Steele, M., & Gallagher, M. (1985). Lipid, kilocalorie, and selected mineral intakes of rural black schoolgirls. *American Journal of Public Health, 75,* 1323–1324.

Steele, M., & Spurgeon, J. (1983). Body size, body form, and nutritional intake of black girls age 9 years living in rural and urban regions of eastern North Carolina. *Growth, 47,* 207–216.

Stehr-Green, P., Farrar, J., Burse, V., Royce, W., & Wohlleb, J. (1988). A survey of measured levels and dietary sources of selected organochlorine pesticide residues and metabolites in human sera from a rural population. *American Journal of Public Health, 78,* 828–830.

Stein, H. (1987). Effects of rural/urban stereotypes in medical education. *High Plains Applied Anthropologist, 7*(1), 11–15.

Stoller, E., & Forster, L. (1992). Patterns of illness behavior among rural elderly: Preliminary results of a health diary study. *Journal of Rural Health, 8,* 13–26.

Sullivan, T., Weinert, C., & Fulton, R. (1993). Living with cancer: Self-identified needs of rural dwellers. *Family & Community Health, 16*(2), 41–49.

Thorson, J., & Powell, F. (1992). Rural and urban elderly construe health differently. *The Journal of Psychology, 126,* 251–260.

Tilden, V. (1985). Issues of conceptualization and measurement of social support in the construction of nursing theory. *Research in Nursing & Health, 8,* 199–206.

U.S. Bureau of the Census. (1987). Statistical abstract of the United States: 1988 (108th ed.). Washington, DC: U.S. Government Printing Office.

U.S. Department of Health and Human Services. (1993). *Aging: Meeting the needs of the rural elderly* (Administration on Aging, No. 365). Washington, DC.: U.S. Government Printing Office.

Van Nostrand, J. (1993). *Common beliefs about the rural elderly: What do national data tell us?* (National Center for Health Statistics, Vital Health Statistics, Vol. 3, No. 28). Washington, DC: U.S. Government Printing Office.

Wagenfeld, M. (1990). Mental health and rural America: A decade review. *Journal of Rural Health, 6,* 507–522.

Wallace, J., & O'Hara, M. (1992). Increases in depressive symptomatology in the rural elderly: Results from a cross-sectional and longitudinal study. *Journal of Abnormal Psychology, 101,* 398–404.

Walters, C., & McHenry, P. (1985). Predictors of life satisfaction among rural and urban employed mothers: A research note. *Journal of Marriage and the Family, 47,* 1067–1071.

Weigel, R., & Weigel, D. (1988). Identifying stressors and coping strategies in two-generation farm families. In R. Marotz-Baden, C. B. Hennon, & T. H. Brubaker (Eds.), *Family in rural America: Stress. adaptation and revitalization* (pp. 216–224). St. Paul, MN: National Council of Family Relations.

Weiler, K., & Buckwalter, K. (1992). Geriatric mental health: Abuse among rural mentally ill. *Journal of Psychosocial Nursing, 30*(9), 32–36.

Weinert, C., & Bender, L. (1993). [Home Care of Rural Cancer Patients in Montana]. Unpublished raw data. Montana State University, College of Nursing, Bozeman, MT.

Weinert, C., & Boik, R. (1993). *MSU Rurality Index: Development and evaluation.* Unpublished manuscript, Montana State University, College of Nursing, Bozeman, MT.

Weinert, C., & Long, K. (1987). Understanding the health care needs of rural families. *Family Relations, 36,* 450–455.

Weinert, C., & Long, K. (1990). Rural families and health care: Refining the knowledge base. *Journal of Marriage and Family Relations, 15*(1&2), 57–75.

Weinert, C., & Long, K. (1991). The theory and research base for rural nursing practice. In A. Bushy (Ed.), *Rural nursing* (Vol. 1, pp 21–38). Newbury Park, CA: Sage.

Weinert, C., & Long, K. (1993). Support systems for spouses of the chronically ill. *Family and Community Health, 16,* 46–54.

Whetstone, W., & Reid, J. (1991). Health promotion of older adults: Perceived barriers. *Journal of Advanced Nursing, 16,* 1343–1349.

Wilhelm, M., & Ridley, C. (1988). Stress and unemployment in rural nonfarm couples: A study of hardships and coping resources. *Family Relations, 37,* 50–54.

Wilson-Ford, V. (1992). Health-protective behaviors of rural black elderly women. *Health and Social Work, 17,* 28–36.

Windley, P., & Scheidt, R. (1983). Service utilization and activity participation arnong psychologically vulnerable and well elderly in rural small towns. *Gerontologist, 23,* 283–287.

Winfree, L., & Griffiths, C. (1983). Social learning and adolescent marijuana use: A trend study of deviant behavior in a rural middle school. *Rural Sociology, 48,* 219–239.

Wright, J., Champagne, F., Dever, G., & Clark, F. (1985). A comparative analysis of rural and urban mortality in Georgia, 1979. *American Journal of Preventive Medicine, 1,* 22–29.

Wright, K. (1993). Management of agricultural injuries and illness. *Nursing Clinics of North America, 23,* 253–266.

Yesalis, C., Lemke, J., Wallace, R., Kohout, F., & Morris, M. (1985). Health status of the rural elderly according to farm history work: The Iowa 65+ rural health study. *Archives of Environmental Health, 40,* 245–253.

Zadinsky, J., & Boettcher, J. (1992). Preventability of infant mortality in a rural community. *Nursing Research, 41,* 223–227.

Zvonkovic, A., Guss, T., & Ladd, L. (1988). Making the most of jobless: Individual and marital features of underemployment. In R. Marotz-Baden, C. Hennon, & T. Brubaker (Eds.), *Family in rural America: Stress, adaptation and revitalization* (pp. 116–125). St. Paul, MN: National Council of Family Relations.

PART II

Research on
Nursing Care Delivery

Chapter 5

Nursing Workload Measurement Systems

SANDRA R. EDWARDSON
SCHOOL OF NURSING
UNIVERSITY OF MINNESOTA

PHYLLIS B. GIOVANNETTI
FACULTY OF NURSING
UNIVERSITY OF ALBERTA

CONTENTS

Workload measurement in nursing is designed to capture the variable nature of the demand for nursing care. Workload measurement systems grew out of a need to predict on a daily basis the number of nurses required to care for in-hospital patients. Historical analysis of the staffing predictions led to the development of fixed and variable staffing patterns. Although many of the systems reviewed are also used to estimate the costs of care provided, it is beyond the scope of this review to evaluate the literature relevant to determining the costs of nursing care (for such reviews, see Edwardson & Giovannetti, 1987; Lampe, 1987; McCloskey, Gardner, & Johnson, 1987; Sovie, 1988). For purposes of this review, a workload measurement system is defined as a method for quantifying nursing activity for staffing purposes. Systems typically include one or more instruments for measuring the time required for direct and indirect nursing care, selected ongoing maintenance functions of the nursing organization, and the personal activities of the nurse. Algorithms are then applied to these measurements to provide an estimate of the number and, in some cases, type of staff necessary to provide the service.

SEARCH PROCEDURE

Major reviews of the literature relevant to nursing workload measurement systems were completed in 1973, 1978 and 1981 (Aydelotte, 1973; Giovannetti, 1978; Young, Giovannetti, Lewison, & Thoms, 1981). This review covers works published between 1977 and December 1992. The search began with three computerized databases: Nursing and Allied Health, Health Planning and Administration, and MEDLINE. Keywords used were patient classification, nursing classification, workload, acuity, and nursing intensity. The search of the databases was supplemented by tracking citations in retrieved articles and by the reviewers' accumulated files and informal knowledge of fugitive literature. No attempt was made to find all relevant dissertations although those known to the reviewers were considered. Notably absent from the published literature were reports of the development and testing of some of the most widely used proprietary systems such as Medicus, M-dax, and GRASP[R].

Had a strict definition of research been used in selecting literature to review, the chapter would have been quite short. Articles related to the description and measurement of nursing workload were included if the work resulted in a product that was subjected to at least a minimal level of systematic testing and whose development was described in sufficient detail to permit evaluation of the methods used. Workload systems were considered relevant if they were designed for nurse staffing regardless of the setting where nursing is practiced. The papers reviewed were categorized into those developed for acute hospitals, long-term care facilities, ambulatory settings, and community settings including public health and home care.

HISTORICAL ANTECEDENTS

Consideration of the relationship between the nursing care time required by patients and the numbers of nursing personnel required can be traced back to the period of Florence Nightingale. Based on the professional judgment of the ward sister, the most seriously ill patients were placed closest to her office to facilitate their observation, whereas patients who could fend for themselves tended to be located at the far end of the large, open wards. One of the first searches for quantitative measures of the demand for nursing care in hospitals was conducted by the National League for Nursing Education (NLNE) (1937). A survey of the practices of 50 selected hospitals in New York revealed that the median number of hours of bedside nursing was 3.4 to 3.5 per patient day. The authors suggested that this figure should be considered a minimum and that further study of the factors essential for organizing and evaluating hospital nursing services was required prior to determining the right number of nursing hours. The League's recommendation appears to have been largely ignored for several decades in that 3.4 to 3.5 hours of care per patient day became a goal for hospitals below the median and a limitation for those that were above. This marked the beginning of global averages as staffing standards (Giovannetti, 1978). Almost 30 years after the NLNE identified the global average, a survey revealed that the standard most commonly accepted for estimating nurse staffing requirements in Canadian hospitals was 3.5 hours of care per patient day (Canadian Nurses Association, 1966).

The work of Connor and others at the Johns Hopkins Hospital is frequently cited as the impetus for the development of systems designed to measure nursing workload and particularly for those systems employing the concepts of classification (Connor, 1960, 1961a, 1961b; Connor, Flagle, Hseih, Preston, & Singer, 1961). Connor developed a three-category classification scheme based on observable physical and emotional care requirements of patients. Through continuous direct care observational studies, an estimate of the nursing care time requirements for patients within each category was provided. A number of other significant findings were revealed by Connor's studies: nursing workload was not a function of gross census but rather the number of patients in each care category, a wide variation in nursing workload existed from day to day, variation in the demand for nursing staff was independent from ward to ward, and the main determinant of nursing workload was the number of class 3 or intensive care patients (Wolfe & Young, 1965a, 1965b). It should be noted that earlier attempts at nursing workload measurement, including both classification and nonclassification schemes, preceded the work of Connor. A number of sources are available for the reader interested in the historical development in the U.S., Canada, and the United Kingdom (Abdellah & Levine,

1965, 1979; Aydelotte, 1973; Baar, Moores & Rhys-Hearn, 1973; Buchan, 1979; Giovannetti, 1978; Young et al., 1981).

TERMINOLOGY/SEMANTIC ISSUES

The terminology employed in reference to workload measurement systems varies widely and has contributed to both misunderstandings and misuse. The term "patient classification system" is frequently used, leading to confusion with many other types of patient classification systems such as Diagnosis Related Groups (DRG), Case Mix Groups (CMG), and Medical Severity of Illness systems. Further, the term is incorrectly used to describe many of the nursing workload measurement systems that do not employ the grouping or classification of patients.

The terms "severity" and "acuity" have also been used to describe nursing workload measurement systems, suggesting a purpose or intent beyond the measurement of nursing care time. Within the health care domain, the terms severity and acuity have a well established meaning, that is, the state of illness or seriousness of the patient's condition. Two early studies by the NLNE (1948, 1949) reported that the patients' degree of illness did not necessarily reflect the intensity of the demand for nursing care. This fact is well recognized by practicing nurses today and has been more recently highlighted in the current debate about the inappropriateness of DRGs and medical severity of illness schemes to represent patients' requirements for nursing care (Jones, 1984). The terms "nursing intensity" and "patient dependency" have frequently been offered as more suitable terms to describe the array of nurse staffing systems, although the preferred term in North America appears to be that of nursing workload measurement systems.

APPROACHES TO WORKLOAD MEASUREMENT

A variety of approaches to the measurement of nursing workload have been developed and although substantial differences exist among the approaches, at minimum they all aim to estimate the total hours of nursing staff required to care for patients. In that the systems were developed primarily to project staffing requirements, most employ a prospective approach to the assessment of patient requirements for nursing care. One notable exception is the Nursing Intensity Index developed by Reitz (1985a, 1985b).

No single source document describing the number of different systems available and/or in use was located. Many systems are developed by vendors and are not fully described in the published literature. Further, many institutions have substantially modified proprietary systems or created their own and details of such systems, if published, remain largely anecdotal and nonresearch based. Early reviews by Abdellah and Levine (1965, 1979), Baar et al. (1973) and Giovannetti (1978) contain examples of a variety of systems but are essentially descriptive in nature. As part of the U.S. Prospective Payment Assessment Commission's evaluation of alternative approaches to Medicare's methods of allocating nursing costs, Cromwell and Harrow (1985) evaluated 14 "of the more prominent systems currently in use" (p. 1-1). Their evaluation, based on secondary published materials supplemented by personal conversations, included the variables or factors used in each system and evidence, if any, of the reliability and validity of each system. The systems reviewed varied significantly in the breadth and depth of activities used to predict nursing resources, leading the reviewers to speculate considerable differences in their ability to estimate nursing needs. Although all of the systems had reportedly undergone some reliability and validity testing, the rigor was highly variable and the published reports generally disappointing, including the widely used GRASP[R] and Medicus systems (pp. 3-19).

Lewis (1989) published a manual containing examples of systems, reported by 35 hospitals and, representing "a cross section of patient classification systems used successfully in hospital nursing departments throughout the United States" (p. 5-1). The information provided in each system was obtained directly from the participating institutions and includes a brief description of the system, including forms used, system evaluation (i.e., reliability and validity), resource and plans for future system requirements. Although the manual provides an interesting account of the experience of the participating institutions, the information is largely anecdotal with insufficient data to evaluate the merits of each system. Most of the facilities reported applications to a wide range of specialty units or note future plans for adaptations to specialty areas. Continued modifications in the systems, computerization and expansion to serve as costing systems were also commonly reported as the focus for future system refinements. Consistent with the findings reported by Cromwell and Harrow (1985), the rigor of reliability and validity testing as reported by the contributors to the Lewis manual was highly variable and generally disappointing. One of the most carefully prepared and thorough analyses of different systems was conducted by Thibault (1990)—an appraisal of the scientific basis of three systems, GRASP[R], Medicus, and PRN, used in the province of Quebec. An important impetus for the evaluation was the finding by O'Brien-Pallas (1987) that substantial differences existed between the three instruments in their predictions of required nursing care hours on the same sample of patients. For the Thibault evaluation, the developers of each of the three systems provided written material in response to an evaluation grid consisting of scientific parameters (e.g., operational definitions, sampling, reliability, and validity) and administrative applications (e.g., uses, application to specialty areas, and components of nursing workload measures). On the basis of the written material, the strengths and weaknesses of the three systems are noted. This review criticizes the developers for lack of evidence about the scientific merit of their instruments and methodologies. The vendors argue, on the other hand, that the data supporting reliability and validity are necessarily user-based. The fact that these and other vendor-developed and implemented systems are widely used throughout North America suggests some degree of acceptance among users. Nonetheless, there is a paucity of evidence attesting to the scientific merit of the systems.

In the United States, it is generally assumed that most hospitals over 50 beds have used or are currently using a workload measurement system and many have had experience with more than one system. A recent survey of 300 randomly selected hospitals in Canada (response rate = 72%) revealed that 67% of the hospitals with greater than 50 beds reported having a workload measurement system in place in one or more clinical setting (O'Brien-Pallas & Cockerill, 1989). The percentage of teaching hospitals and nonteaching hospitals over 300 beds using a system was reported to be over 80%. Comparable statistics from the United Kingdom were not identified; however, a review of over 50 published and unpublished works in Great Britain from 1963–1975 in the area of patient–nurse dependency suggest a significant level of interest and activity (Wilson-Barnett, 1978).

Types of Workload Measurement Systems

The proliferation of workload measurement systems coupled with the absence of literature describing the details of the system makes it difficult to clarify the distinctions between the systems. Giovannetti (1984) described three major approaches: patient profiles, critical indicators of care, and nursing task documents. Profile instruments are characterized by broad descriptions of the characteristics of a typical patient in each category and are commonly referred to as "prototype evaluations" (Abdellah & Levine, 1979). The actual characteristics of the patient are compared with those described in the profiles and the patient is then designated as belonging to the category that most closely matches the profile or prototype description. Prototype descriptions are frequently adjusted for specialty units such as pediatrics, surgery, oncology, and so on. All profile instruments employ the concepts of classification although they differ in the precision of the prototypical statements. Many of the earliest workload measurement systems were of this type but were notably general in the descriptors used. More recent systems [e.g., Allocation Resource Identification and Costing (ARIC)] have employed statistical means for developing the prototypical statements (Giovannetti & Johnson, 1990). It should be noted that the DRG system, although not a nursing workload measurement system, is an example of the prototype approach.

The critical indicators approach is possibly the most common and employs the listing of specific elements of care and/or indicators representing clusters of care activities. Among the elements selected are those that are considered to correlate most highly with varying amounts of nursing care time required by patients. Indicators reflecting specific therapeutic needs such as assistance with feeding, bathing, and ambulation have through time demonstrated their usefulness in distinguishing patients who require extensive nursing care time from those requiring minimal nursing care time and are almost universally included in one form or another. Other indicators such as patient condition (e.g., unconscious); patient state (e.g., blind); specific nursing activities (e.g., complex dressing change) and statements reflecting the emotional and teaching needs of patients are prevalent. The number, the nature and the specificity of indicators vary widely and as suggested by Hanson (1979), the inclusion of indicators is based not only on their contribution to the statistical validity of the classification scheme, but on their contribution to user acceptability and face validity. These schemes are also known as factor evaluation systems (Abdellah & Levine, 1979) and all employ the principles of categorization or grouping. Ratings on each individual patient characteristic or element of care (factor) are combined for an overall rating, which, when compared to a set of decision rules, identifies the appropriate care category. The systems developed by Connor (1960) and Medicus are classic examples of this approach. As is the case with the prototype systems, the critical indicators selected are frequently modified to reflect different clinical specialties.

The naming of the critical indicators and the number of critical indicators are perhaps the two most obvious features that differentiate workload measurement systems of this type. No evidence was found to suggest that the types of indicators (e.g., patient states, care procedures) or the number of indicators (e.g., less than 10 or more than 40) have a bearing on the validity of the workload measurement system. Nonetheless, most of the anecdotal (descriptive) literature on workload measurement systems, with varying degrees of scholarliness, argue for the merits of one system over another essentially on the selection of the labels and the numbers of indicators.

The third approach to the development of workload measurement systems, nursing task documents, does not rely on the creation of patient groups or categories. Systems of this type employ a listing of direct care nursing tasks or activities specific to each clinical specialty. Each task or activity is associated with a value representing the time required to carry out the activity or a relative value representing time coefficients. Patients are independently assessed on the basis of their need for each task or activity and the outcomes of the assessment yields a unique care time for each patient. Similar to the factor-evalu-

CARL A. RUDISILL LIBRARY
LENOIR-RHYNE COLLEGE

ation schemes, task documents differ with respect to the number of tasks cited. The GRASP^R system works on the principle that 40 to 50 direct care activities account for 85% of the direct care time on medical/surgical units. Some versions of PRN contain over 200 tasks (Thibault, 1990).

Establishing Hours of Care

A variety of approaches ranging from estimates derived from expert opinion to real-time values derived from extensive timing studies have been used to establish time coefficients for workload measurement systems. A number of approaches are unique to the type of workload measurement system employed, whereas others can be applied to all types. The literature is replete with references to the general approaches used for quantifying the workload measurement systems although details sufficient to establish the accuracy of the coefficients are lacking.

All workload measurement systems that employ the concept of grouping or classification, whether of the profile or critical indicator type, seek to provide an average care time per patient category. The derivation of average care time differs significantly. For example, the nursing hours per patient day (NHPPD) assigned to each of the five-category prototype oncology system reported by Arenth (1985) were originally derived from standard NHPPD reported in the literature coupled with nurses' estimates of the nursing resources required for each level and retrospective review of the institutional data. Johnson (1984) described a prototype system that was quantified through self-recording methods of staff representing their estimates of the average care time required for patients in each of the four categories. A fifth category (intensive care) was determined a priori to require continuous care and therefore was exempt from further estimation. Other prototype systems have established hours of care retrospectively through either continuous or intermittent (sampling) observational techniques (Lewis, 1989). Presumably, if significant differences in care times between groups are not revealed, the criteria for establishing the groups are reevaluated.

It should be noted that quantification techniques generally take into account the time required for both the direct and indirect care as described in the classification or tasking document as well as the nondirect care components associated with staffing a unit. This latter determination is essential to the aim of all of the systems, that of determining the number of nurses required per shift or 24-hour period (U.S. Department of Health, Education, and Welfare, 1978).

Quantification methods employed with tasking documents are less variable than those applied to prototype and factor-evaluation systems, no doubt due to the nature of the instruments. Essentially they employ the use of real times, standard times, or average times per procedure or task. The derivation of these times extends from simple estimation procedures to extensive data from observational studies. The underlying assumption of tasking documents is that the sum of the parts (discrete nursing tasks) is equal to the whole. As previously noted, tasking documents differ considerably in the precision used to define the discrete tasks and thus range from systems employing less than 50 items to those with over 200.

Comparability of Systems

The comparability of the different workload measurement systems has received limited attention in the literature. Indeed, until recently there appears to have been a general acceptance that all systems were equivalent given that reliability coefficients were acceptable and validity assessments were conducted from time to time. Further, because staffing levels are not only a function of patients' requirements for care but of other variables such as the physical layout and design of units, physician practices and staffing mixes, emphasis has been placed on the development of care times unique to each facility and in many cases, to each unit within a facility (Young et al., 1981). Two early attempts at comparability focused on the equivalence of the categories of care and yielded similar findings. Roehrl (1979) reported moderate to high correlations in the dispersion of patients into care categories using three factor evaluation instruments. Based on the findings, she argued for selection of the system most preferred by the nursing staff. Schroeder, Rhodes, and Shields (1984) came to the same conclusions in their comparison of two systems. Both investigations were based on small samples and, as previously noted, considered only the assignment of the category of care.

The seminal work of O'Brien-Pallas, Cockerill, and Leatt (1991) has shed new light on the question of comparability. In her doctoral dissertation, O'Brien-Pallas (1987) reported significant differences in staffing estimates. Two of the systems were tasking documents: PRN 76 with 154 care activities and GRASP[R] with 50 activities for the ICU version and 35 for the non-ICU version. Medicus was the third instrument tested and, although technically referred to as a factor-evaluation instrument, the use of relative weights for the 37 indicators was, in the view of the investigator, sufficient justification for comparison as a tasking document. The GRASP[R] system was already in place in the 1000-bed hospital selected for the study. Medicus and PRN developers were responsible for implementation of their systems including recalibration of time estimates on the seven study units, which included both ICU and non-ICU units. The hypothesis that PRN 76 would predict more direct care hours than GRASP[R] or Medicus was confirmed. There were no differences between Medicus and GRASP[R] in total hours, but there were significant differences among all systems at the unit level. All three systems were found to be highly correlated.

A replication of this study in a second hospital produced essentially the same findings using five workload measurement systems: PRN 76, PRN 80, Medicus, GRASP[R], and NISS (O'Brien-Pallas et al., 1991). Differences as great as 4.53 hours per day for the same patient were observed. The high correlations between the systems led the investigators to develop relational statements between the systems for the purposes of comparing nursing care costs. The findings of these two studies are significant in that all systems studied were considered to yield time estimates specifically validated for the same study units and interrater reliability testing was high (91%–98%) during data collection. For the five instruments tested in the replication study, the findings generally revealed that the greater the number of items, the higher the estimates of nursing care time.

The work of Phillips, Castorr, Prescott, and Soeken (1992) is also of significance to the question of comparability. Their investigation focused on the relationship between the workload predictions of Medicus, GRASP[R], and PINI (Patient Intensity Nursing Index). The sample consisted of patient ratings from 24 clinical units representing four hospitals. Concurrent ratings were obtained using PINI and Medicus (1827 patients) and using PINI and GRASP[R] (1117 patients). Although PINI was developed as a measure of nursing costs and the purpose of the study was to investigate the adequacy of Medicus and GRASP[R] as measures of costs, the findings support those of the previous investigations, namely, that although highly correlated, the comparability of nursing workload measures should not be assumed.

Adaptations to Specialty Areas

Much of the workload measurement system development in the last decade has been devoted to the adaptation and/or modification of systems for specialty areas. Although many of the major systems claim to be applicable to a variety of specialty areas, potential users appear to be reluctant to accept such claims. The descriptive literature is replete with accounts of modifications and adjustments for specialty areas. The two areas that have been most extensively involved in development or major modifications are psychiatry and intensive care. Several unique psychiatric instruments have been published employing both the factor evaluation and tasking document approaches (Eklof & Qu, 1986; Morath, Fleischmann, & Boggs, 1989; Pardue & Dick, 1986; Ringerman & Luz, 1990; Schroeder, Washington, Deering, & Coyne, 1986). Two psychiatric workload measurement systems are direct adaptations of GRASP[R] (Ehrman, 1987; Thomas & Moses, 1986).

Critical care instrument development includes the Therapeutic Intervention Scoring System (TISS) and modifications of the San Joachin system (Ambutas, 1987; 1988; Burger & Schmitt, 1982; Cullen, Civetta, Briggs, & Ferrara, 1974; Keene & Cullen, 1983; Niemeier & Reed, 1985). As with the vast majority of published materials on workload measurement systems, sufficient information on the development of the instrument, including the quantification approach, was lacking.

Long-Term Care

In long-term care, there has been less interest in workload measurement systems than in the application of classification schemes to place individuals in the most appropriate care option. Given the high cost of nursing home care, most work has concentrated on identifying whether or not nursing home care is required and, if so, what level of care is needed. Case-mix systems for setting payment rates are based either on service intensity or clusters of patient characteristics (Hogan & Smith, 1987). Information about the required level of care is important for determining nurse staffing over a period of time but is less useful for making intermediate and short-term decisions.

In her historical analysis of the field, Boondas (1991) identified a growing consensus that assessment should be based on impairment and disability rather than medical diagnosis. Most descriptions of the field confirm the importance of functional status and impairment, but also include variables related to the individual's medical condition (Densen & Jones, 1976; Katz, Hedrick, & Henderson, 1979; Leatt, Bay, & Stinson, 1981; Mitty, 1987).

On the whole, classification systems used in long-term care were developed using more sophisticated methods than those for other areas of care. Bay, Leatt, and Stinson (1983) developed a system using functional level, disease category, risk factors, and health indices. Beginning with traditional criterion-related validity (using evaluations of an independent panel as the criterion), they applied stepwise discriminant analysis and binary cluster analysis in an iterative process, alternating classification and modification of criterion groups until the membership of each type stabilized.

Cavaiola and Young (1980) used functional status, behavioral status, and medically defined conditions as indicators and subjected them to logistic function modeling, fitting three simultaneous equations to predict the prior probability that a patient required one of three levels of care. Then backward elimination with ordinary multiple linear regression was performed in order to identify a subset of variables useful for grouping patients into categories with similar care needs. Having grouped the patients by care needs, the investigators then used mathematical programming strategies to develop alternate staffing strategies.

The Resource Utilization Groups (RUGs) system, widely used as a case-mix measure for long-term care patients in the U.S., uses nursing care time as the dependent variable (Fries & Cooney, 1985). Hogan and Smith (1987) used classifications of patients by the RUGs system as the criterion against which to validate their independently developed classification system.

The Alberta Health Long-Term Care study (Semradek et al., 1988) had the dual purposes of providing information for staffing and a case-mix measure for funding long-term care facilities. An expert panel developed a classification system by defining and combining care indicators. The categories developed were verified against empirical standards using self-reported staff activity data from a stratified sample of 11 facilities. Careful, repeated measurements of reliability were taken followed by remedial work until reliability reached an acceptable level. Patient care indicators were selected on the basis of their ability to increase explained variance. The most powerful predictors were used to develop a set of prototype statements, one for each of the seven levels of care. The classification scheme was then subjected to four tests: homogeneity, discriminability, ordinality, and predictive validity.

In summary, most classification systems in long-term care can be labeled more appropriately as case mix systems designed to identify the appropriate care option and reimbursement level rather than to facilitate variable staffing. Development and validation methods used for long-term care systems have tended to be much more sophisticated than those used for acute care systems. Historically the nursing intensity and day-to-day changes in care requirements for long-term care clients have been lower than that of acute care patients. This has meant that managers have not faced the wide variations in care requirements from one day to the next and have been able to function with less measurement precision. Current trends toward greater nursing intensity in long-term care may change that and render long-term care similar to acute care a decade ago. If so, the need for workload measurement systems sensitive to frequent changes in care requirements may become necessary in long-term care as well.

Community Health

Two important attempts to describe the work of community and home health nursing are the Omaha Classification Scheme (Martin, 1982; Simmons, 1980) and the nursing intervention taxonomy study (Saba, O'Hare, Zuckerman, Boondas, Levine, & Oatway, 1991). The Omaha system classifies client problems using 38 problem labels divided into four domains: environmental, psychosocial, physiological, and health behavior (Martin, 1982; Simmons, 1980). In use, the nurse identifies appropriate expected outcomes and outcome criteria for existing problems. The developers have not reported quantification of the system for staffing purposes but others have used the taxonomy to measure staffing needs, usually in terms of the number of visits required.

Peters (1988) built on the Omaha system in developing the Community Health Intensity Rating Scale (CHIRS) for predicting resource consumption according to the four domains of the Omaha system. The test of the scale showed overall interrater agreement of 77%. Concurrent validity was estimated by correlating CHIRS with the number of nursing visits ($r = .39$) and a functional limitation score on the Health Status Scale ($r = .38$).

Hays (1992) compared the ability of the CHIRS and nursing diagnoses for explaining the variance of direct hours of nursing care in the home. CHIRS explained only 10% of the variance, whereas nursing diagnoses explained between 34% and 39%. But as Hays noted, the presence or absence of diagnoses as an indicator is difficult both conceptually and practically and ventured that a multivariate predictor set may produce more satisfactory results.

Helberg (1989) found the Omaha system omitted necessary assessment and intervention indicators and was too long for staff nurses to be proficient. She developed a 26-item classification index using a review of the literature and expert opinion to identify the indicators of assessment and intervention needs. Interrater agreement was evaluated by using case vignettes and observation of home visits. The instrument was quantified by using the mean time spent on each activity as observed by the investigator and reported by the practicing nurse.

As part of a home health care classification project, Saba and associates (1991) developed a taxonomy of nursing interventions used in home health care. A total of 640 unique nursing interventions clustered into 60 major nursing service categories were derived from a textual analysis of 1000 cases. Finally, 20 discrete home health care components were derived from statistical analysis to form a coding structure. Uses of the taxonomy for investigating resource use in home health care are forthcoming.

Several more traditional classification studies designed to measure the need for nursing services have also been reported. Churness, Kleffel, and Onodera (1991) conducted a carefully designed three-phase study to create and test a factor evaluation instrument. Reliability was assessed using interrater agreement and predictive validity was measured using length of home visits as the criterion.

Allen, Easley, and Storfjell (1986) developed a method using a matrix that cross-tabulated the number of home visits required by a client over a period of time with a four-level determination of case difficulty. Because the scale's measurement properties were not reported, Albrecht (1991) tested the reliability and validity of both the factor and prototype versions of the Easley-Storfjell (ES) instrument using a random sample of 30 patient records. Although the correlation between the factor and prototype versions of the scale was significant (.75), both interrater reliability (using Kendall's coefficient of concordance, W) and intrarater reliability (using Spearman rank correlation, r_s) were higher for the factor (W = .57 and r_s = .83, respectively) than the prototype version (W = .48 and r_s = .61). Concurrent validity of the physical care variable of the instrument was assessed against the Katz Activities of Daily Living (ADL) scale, producing a Kendall's tau correlation of .55 and Spearman rank correlation of .64.

A number of studies were reported that used patient classification as a variable to describe or forecast the use of resources in home care. Harris, Santoferraro, and Silva (1985) used a combination of quality assurance and medical diagnostic information to identify costs. They built on the work of Daubert (1979), who had developed the Rehabilitation Potential Patient Classification System to group patients on admission to the visiting nurses association into one of five categories based on their rehabilitation potential. Care objectives were identified for each group. Harris et al., (1985) used the Daubert system to create a quality management system. By combining the quality data with information on each patient's major diagnostic category, they were able to describe the intensity and cost of services for meaningful patient groups.

Several forecasting attempts have been reported. Ballard and McNamara (1983) found the Health Status Scale (HSS) to explain more variance than any other variable in stepwise multiple regression of nursing visits per day and total agency visits per day on independent variables. The HHS is an 18-item four-point scale (no, minor, moderate, serious problem) with indicators of sensory, communication, ADLs, continence, behavior, and skin as variables.

Edwardson and Nardone (1990) tested the usefulness of the Dependency at Discharge Instrument for predicting resource use in home care. The factor type instrument assesses patients on four variables: activity/mobility, bathing/hygiene, procedures, and signs/symptom monitoring. It was found to have good internal consistency and interrater reliability and modest criterion-related validity (using the number of nurse visits, number of home health aide visits and length of enrollment). It appeared to be less valid for public health and for-profit agencies than for a hospital-affiliated agency.

Although Rookes' (1982) report of her attempt to identify a reasonable caseload for health visitors in England provides no empirical results, it is included here because it used a unique method for determining workload. A health visitor was selected who was judged to have an optimal caseload. Then the nature of the cases and distribution of time among activities for the referent caseload were analyzed and verified against five other representative caseloads.

To summarize the work in community health, two major taxonomies have concentrated on describing and documenting the care needs of clients. These taxonomies have been viewed as promising sources of indicators for workload measurement systems. At least one investigator (Helberg, 1989) has found the taxonomic approach to be too detailed and cumbersome while missing some of the assessment and intervention activities that influence the amount of time required to provide care. Those investigators who have used more traditional development approaches have differed in what should be considered the dependent variable: number of visits, length of visits, or length of episode of care. There seems to be a desire for a data system that combines documentation of care given with workload determination. A next step may be for the two streams of work to converge to address this goal.

Ambulatory

There are several features of ambulatory care that make workload measurement different than in acute care. These include the episodic nature and unclear boundaries of the treatment period, unclear and variable requirements for nursing, minimal limits on workload capacity, patient rather than provider control of timing, and the fact that ambulatory nursing may not be managed by nurses (Hastings, 1987). Hoffman and Wakefield (1986) also mentioned the fact that different nursing technologies are employed; ambulatory staffing must be based on information gathered retrospectively; and there is a high likelihood of additional walk-ins, overbookings, broken appointments, and modifications necessary because of physician scheduling preferences.

Ambulatory patients have been classified by medical diagnosis, nursing care requirements, and purpose of visit. Fetter, Averill, Lichtenstein, and Freeman (1984) developed a DRG-like system for ambulatory care that groups patients by characteristics that predict the expenditure of provider time. Using the AUTOGRP grouper technique used for developing the DRGs, iso-resource categories were uncovered by combining information about medical diagnosis, presenting problem, reason for visit, visit type, and patient age. No studies investigating the relevance of this method for describing the use of nursing resources was uncovered, but it would seem to be a potentially fruitful area of investigation.

The single most important work for measuring nursing workload in ambulatory care was that completed by Verran (1986a, 1986b). Using Delphi techniques, she developed a taxonomy of 44 nursing activities grouped into six responsibility areas. From this taxonomy, she constructed a factor evaluation instrument, the Ambulatory Care Client Classification Instrument (ACCCI). She tested the validity of the instrument by its ability to capture the complexity of care provided as measured by a subjective complexity rating instrument developed using modified magnitude estimation techniques. Verran proposed a novel method for establishing interrater reliability, one of the more vexing problems in developing classification systems for ambulatory care. Audiotapes of reports on patients were independently rated by the raters trained in using the ACCCI.

After Verran established the utility of the taxonomy for creating meaningful categories of ambulatory patients, Miller and Folse (1989) and Johnson (1989) took the work one step further and described how the hours of care required by patients in each category can be quantified. Unfortunately neither report provided evidence for the reliability and validity of the classification procedure. Joseph (1990) combined Verran's taxonomy with GRASP^R categorizations and a work-sampling instrument to study the distribution of activities among direct, indirect, unit-related, personal, and other tasks and between RN and LVN/NA staff. Although useful as a method for defining staff mix, the method did not include the quantification necessary to permit use for variable staffing.

Hastings and Muir-Nash (1989) revised Verran's taxonomy by sorting the activities into the four phases of nursing care (assessment, planning, intervention, and evaluation). They further described the intervention phase by using Orem's categories of acting, guiding, supporting, providing, and teaching. As a result, they obtained a list of 61 ambulatory care nursing activities grouped into nine responsibility areas. Content validation revealed that, with three exceptions, all activities were confirmed as components of nursing practice in ambulatory care by 50% or more of the 33 managers who served as judges.

Parrinello, Brenner, and Vallone (1988) adapted the ACCCI to their institution and assigned institution-specific weights using Delphi techniques. In application, interrater agreement and overall predictive validity (estimated by the association between actual nursing time as reported by the staff and intensity scores) were high. Intensity scores explained 68% of variance in reported nursing care time. When the data were disaggregated according to provider type, nursing care time and intensity scores showed considerable within-group variability. The investigators concluded that mean care times for visits based on provider type may not be a useful figure to determine daily staffing levels. But when used with volume, it may be useful in examining the aggregate support required and in costing out support provided.

Using a similar strategy to tailor the Verran taxonomy, Shade and Austin (1992) also achieved high interrater agreement. But they computed a variance index (predicted/actual care hours) that ranged from .23 to 3.40 for the various clinics, suggesting the need for additional precision of measurement.

Cohen, Arnold, Brown, and Brooten (1991) applied the ACCCI to the follow-up of low birthweight infants after hospital discharge. They were able to capture all interventions listed in patient records and achieved high interrater reliability (90%). Although they did not use the classification for staffing or cost identification, that could be a future application.

A nonclassificatory example of workload measurement is that of Genovich-Richards and Tracy (1984). Total visit time was regressed on tasks performed (present or absent) to estimate time required for each activity. The intercept of the model was defined to be the time spent on all tasks not recorded. Care activities were grouped into check-in, examination room, and check-out functions. The proportion of variance explained by check-in functions (.92) was much higher than that for examination room (.64), and check-out functions (.39).

The taxonomic approach to identifying critical indicators appears to have been more successful in ambulatory care than in community health. This may be because the Verran taxonomy is one of interventions rather than client characteristics. The volatility and open-endedness of ambulatory care present unique challenges to those developing workload measurement systems. Daily assessment of workload can become extremely cumbersome because of the sheer volume of patients seen. At the same time, the information gathered has less usefulness for predicting tomorrow's staffing requirements because of the extreme variability in demand in many facilities. The search for valid yet practical methods of workload measurement will need to continue.

MEASUREMENT ISSUES

Classification

The task of developing work measurement strategies for nurse staffing requires a method for identifying the variables or critical indicators important in predicting the type and/or amount of nursing care time required. Traditionally these variables have been used to divide patients into isogroups with respect to need for care. More recently additive models that sum either the time or a time-based weight associated with each variable have become popular.

Most of the studies reported in this review have selected variables or indicators without regard to a theoretical base. The selection of classification variables represents an attempt to recognize patterns. A large number of features of the care process are measured and then techniques are used to reduce the number of variables to the lowest number necessary to provide sufficient information to perform the classification task (Cavailoa, 1975). Many classification systems use information about needs for bathing, feeding, ambulation, observation, special treatments, and psychosocial support and teaching (Aydelotte, 1973). Although these few variables are clearly not sufficient to describe or explain the work of the nurse, they have been found sufficient for predicting with acceptable accuracy the nursing care requirements in some future time.

Recently workload measurement systems that include almost all of the activities performed by nurses have become very popular because of a belief that including more variables will provide greater adequacy. The assumption underlying this total enumeration approach is that the whole of nursing care is equal to the sum of its parts (DeGroot, 1989). Giovannetti (1984) argued that this assumption is not valid because nursing care is not delivered at a constant rate throughout a shift. Furthermore, the simultaneous performance of two or more activities (e.g., assessment of consciousness while positioning a patient) can lead to overestimates when times required for individual care activities are simply summed.

Some have argued against utilitarian approaches to identifying critical indicators. Haas (1988) feared that when patient classification systems are not grounded in a theory explaining the work of nursing, they have a way of limiting the scope of nursing. Donnelly (1981) proposed the domains of the Roy model (physiological, psychological, sociological, cultural, and spiritual) as a theoretical basis for patient classification, adding teaching and discharge planning activities. Others have proposed using nursing diagnoses (Halloran, 1985; Karshmer, 1991) or problems encountered by patients (Peters, 1987, 1988).

If the only purpose of workload measurement systems is to predict nursing care requirements in the future, the utilitarian approach would seem to be entirely acceptable. If, on the other hand, users are going to continue to expect that the systems should be useful for describing and documenting patient care as well, it may be advisable to use a more theoretical approach.

Quantification

There are two types of quantification required in measuring nursing workload: the amount of time required for patient-specific care activities and the amount required for all other work. Expert opinion is widely used to establish the time required to perform specific care activities or to care for patients in different categories. Studies testing the accuracy of these estimates are rare.

For systems that use additive models, time studies are used to measure the amount of time spent in performing a specific care activity in the patient's presence and, in most cases, the preparatory, clean-up and documentation work as well. Methods-Time Measurement-Universal Analyzing System (MTM-UAS) is the most reductionistic method for establishing standard care times. It is based on the premise that work can be divided into small elements, times established for each, and then combined to determine the time required for the total task (Lindner, 1989). The description for preparing injectable medications, for example, includes 40 steps beginning with "get and hold syringe" and ending with "get and place trash." Lindner argued that the method eliminates the problem of work pace encountered in work sampling, permits comparison of different methods for performing a job, and is faster to apply, is more accurate, and credible. In applying the method to nursing, however, he encountered problems because of the variability of patients and the fact that time is governed by the patient, not the nurse.

Work sampling is the dominant method for validating the time associated with patient care categories and for quantifying the proportion of time the nurse spends in direct and indirect care and in unit-related and personal activities. Work sampling is based on the proposition that when personnel are randomly observed performing activities, the relative frequency of an activity is highly correlated with the proportion of time spent on the activity. Because staffing levels at the time of work sampling become the de facto staffing standard, it must be assumed that the staffing levels are acceptable for achieving the desired level of quality.

There are two issues involved in work sampling: the method for recording observations and the frequency of observations. Many investigators (e.g., Hagerty, Chang, & Spengler, 1985) use self-logging of activities to estimate time. Although less expensive than employing work sampling observers, self-logging carries the risk of conscious or unconscious misrepresentation of activities.

Most work sampling studies observe each member of the nursing staff every 15 minutes, with the observer going from one nurse to the next; the observer records what the nurse is doing and which patient is being cared for, if any. Variations include random selection of time intervals and randomly altering the order in which nurses are observed. Simulation studies by Flowerdew and Malin (1963) led them to conclude that fixed interval sampling can give more accurate results than random sampling when a sampling interval is shorter than the shortest elements that can be used. This permits the largest sample size of nursing activity per day of observation while limiting the number of observation days to a practical number. Work measurement at 1-minute intervals, for example, produces 480 observations per nurse per day. Twenty days of observation would produce 9600 observations per nurse and provides accuracy within +/– 3.5% at a 95% confidence level (Maynard, 1971).

Reliability

Regardless of how the care needs are assessed and patients are grouped, reliability of measurement is a major concern. Because workload measurement systems are designed to be used by many nurses, it is important that the nurses be consistent in their measurement in order to ensure accuracy.

Of the three major types of reliability (stability, homogeneity, and equivalence), most studies reported in the literature have used interrater reliability (a measure of equivalence) evaluated as a simple percentage of agreement among staff nurses and an expert classifier. Sources of error in interrater reliability can occur at all steps in the measurement process: (a) disagreement on definition of assessment items, (b) failure to follow instructions in arriving at summary items, (c) failure to follow instructions in assigning a final classification, and (d) use of clinical judgment rather than objective criteria (McKenzie, 1991). Agreement was lower when assessment items were global in nature and when judgment was required to integrate data across assessment items.

Chance agreement in estimates of interrater agreement increases as the number of categories decreases and increases if the percentage of items evaluated by the users is high or low (Jennings, Rea, Antopol, & Carty, 1989). To control for the possibility of chance agreement, some have advocated the use of the Kappa (K) statistic to give a measure of the non-chance agreements (Soeken & Prescott, 1986). Overall interrater agreement of 90% is generally considered acceptable (Giovannetti, 1984). Others have proposed the use of analysis of variance as a more powerful and precise measure of interrater agreement (Bigbee, Collins, & Deeds, 1992).

Although interrater agreement about the final classification decision is usually sufficient for day-to-day monitoring of workload measurement systems, it is sometimes wise to evaluate agreement on items used to arrive at the classification decision as well. This is particularly true during the development of a system and in investigating the causes for unsatisfactory reliability. When more than one unit in a facility uses the same instrument, it is necessary to establish inter-unit agreement as well to permit meaningful comparisons of units.

One study comparing nonnursing classification systems evaluated reliability in terms of reduction in variance and by using a coefficient of variance (CV) from the mean of the resource-use variable. The authors argued that the CV, as a measure of dispersion around the mean, is analogous to a confidence interval or simple linear regression (Charbonneau et al., 1988).

The question of whether or not interrater agreement is an adequate technique for evaluating reliability seems to turn on the level of precision necessary. Because workload measurement systems are usually built as an adjunct rather than a substitute for the judgment of a manager, interrater agreement should provide an adequate level of precision in most cases. If, however, the system is to be used for purposes demanding the highest possible precision, then alternate reliability estimation techniques may be indicated.

Validity

Validity of workload measurement systems cannot be addressed without first answering the question of valid for what purpose. Originally patient classification systems for nurse staffing were designed to provide quick and accurate predictions of staffing needs for one or more shifts into the future. As such, classification variables selected are those that are objective, readily available, and statistically powerful as predictors. This minimal set usually included bathing, feeding, ambulation, treatment, and teaching requirements. Lacking an appreciation of the difference between variables that correlate with workload and variables that describe or explain the work of nursing, many have objected to the "taskiness" of these indicators and the omission of activities reflecting the cognitive and discretionary aspects of nursing. Others have sought to combine documentation (charting) and workload measurement systems for greater efficiency and to provide information for medical-legal and cost identification purposes as well. For purposes of this review, validity of workload measurement will be considered in terms of the original meaning, that is, as a statistically powerful predictor of future workload.

Validity of workload measurement systems is generally assessed at the time a system is implemented in a setting. Rapid changes in technology and nursing practices together with frequent reconfiguration of nursing units mean that care activities and their associated times also change rapidly producing a major problem for maintaining validity.

Content validation, in which clinical experts are enlisted to identify or verify the care activities most important for the care of a group of patients, is the most common validation method used. Common techniques for generating lists of activities include brainstorming, nominal group process (Trivedi, 1982), Delphi techniques (Verran, 1981), and Q-sort (Gorham, 1962). Hsiao, Braun, Yntema, and Becker (1988) conceived and verified physician work as having four dimensions: time, mental effort and judgment, technical skill and physical effort, and psychological stress. They estimated the amount of work and time required for services listed in current physician procedural terminology with magnitude estimation; they used a ratio scale of values with magnitudes greater or less than a referent procedure. This method would seem to be directly applicable to consensus estimates of nursing work as well and should be tested.

Soeken and Prescott (1991) employed factor analysis to evaluate the construct validity of the Patient Intensity for Nursing Index. It does not appear that this index has yet been used for estimating staffing requirements, however.

The face validity provided by content validation techniques is important if staff nurses who are not familiar with the conceptual base for classification systems are to have sufficient faith in the measurement to apply the system accurately. The authors' experience suggests that the care activities most salient to nurses are those that require the greatest expenditure of time or effort such as crisis events. Although these activities consume a large amount of resources when they occur, they tend to be relatively rare and not very powerful for predicting the need for care for the bulk of patients. For this reason, content validation (especially face validity) is probably necessary but not sufficient; the validity of care indicators identified by content experts should be evaluated carefully by other methods, such as predictive validity, as well.

Trivedi (1979) used Automatic Interaction Detector, a forerunner of the AUTOGRP analytic system used to develop DRGs, to identify variables necessary to divide patients into groups defined by head nurse judgments. He found that only a few patient classification variables were necessary and that different sets of variables were essential for different shifts on the same unit.

There are a few reports of the use of concurrent validation in which the workload instrument being evaluated is compared to another more established instrument (e.g., O'Brien-Pallas et al., 1991). Williams and Murphy (1979) proposed staffing adequacy as judged by an experienced head or charge nurse as an appropriate criterion. This method rests on the assumption that an experienced nurse manager is a finely tuned measurement instrument, an assumption readily accepted by most nurses but less acceptable to skeptical policy makers outside of nursing. Charbonneau and associates (1988) evaluated construct validity by attempting to produce a monotonic stratification of the resource use variable by ordinal rank.

Logically, if the purpose of workload measurement is to forecast workload for some time in the future, then the most important evidence of validity is predictive validity. Predictive validity is usually established during implementation of a system by comparing the workload predicted by the system with the actual workload observed by time studies. There were three reports in which predictive validity was established by comparing forecasted workload with another retrospective measurement of workload at the end of the period for which the forecast was made (Edwardson, Bahr, & Serote, 1990; Giovannetti & Johnson, 1990; Whitney & Killien, 1987).

Conclusions and Directions for Future Research

Over the past 30 years the literature has been replete with articles, books, and monographs devoted to the topic of nurse staffing. With few exceptions, the answer to the perennial question, . . . how to identify the "right" level of staffing, has been the implementation of patient classification, or more appropriately entitled, nursing workload measurement systems. The promise of the systems was compelling: a more "scientific" approach to replace the subjective (and thus considered biased) judgment of a nurse. Also compelling was the underlying assumption that such systems would lead to the efficient utilization of nursing resources. Thirty years later, little attention has been paid to the fact that a significant portion of nurses' time continues to be spent in nondirect patient care activities many of which do not require the skills and knowledge of nurses.

The number of uniquely different systems developed over the past 30 years is not known although it is assumed to be relatively small. Many systems are replicas of one another, differing only in title, print size, and/or semantics. The extent of implementation is also not known although it is assumed that most hospitals have had experience with one or more systems. Indeed a disturbing finding in the literature is the frequency with which major health care facilities have changed from one system to another with some implementing and discarding three or four different systems over the span of just a few years. This suggests a continuing yet disappointing search for the right system.

The fundamental test of the utility of WMS has been on the basis of their ability to predict nursing workload in the short term, that is, the next shift or 24-hour period. For the most part and in the immediate postimplementation phase, they have proven to be quite satisfactory. With the continued rapid changes in the complexity of both the care required and the settings where care is provided, there is some question about the ability of the systems to provide appropriate long-term staffing information. It would appear that what is behind the continual search for new systems is their lack of stability over time. The systems are in almost constant need of revalidation. Although some users appear to be prepared to monitor validity on an ongoing basis, there is evidence that many are not, leading to inappropriate application and lack of support by nurses. Serious charges of the deprofessionalization of nursing and the deskilling and routinization of nurses' work have all been attributed to the use of the systems (Campbell, 1988; Storch & Stinson, 1988).

After three decades of experience with workload measurement systems, some interesting questions can be raised. Have the implementation of staffing methodologies affectively altered the level of staffing within facilities or have predetermined staffing levels altered the outcome of the workload measurement systems? What, if any, effect have workload measurement systems had on the quality of care? Do the results of a workload measurement system depart significantly from the professional judgment of practicing nurses? Have workload measurement systems resulted in an improvement in the utilization of nursing personnel?

Another fundamental question to be asked is the validity of workload measurement systems as a proxy for nursing costs. As noted in the beginning of this review, many of the systems are also used to predict the costs of care provided. Although the topic of costs was beyond the scope of this chapter, it is recognized that determination of the costs of nursing care has become an essential question for all nurse managers.

It would appear that current trends brought on by the Prospective Payment era will significantly alter the nature and function of workload measurement systems. The argument advanced is that by identifying data elements derived from a meaningful conceptual model of nursing practice, measurement of nursing work cannot only be described consistently and validly across institutions, but estimating workload can become a by-product of a multiuse data set rather than a single-purpose entity. Attention could appropriately be refocused on the evaluation of nursing practices to yield information on the efficacy of nursing care.

In conclusion, research related to staffing predictions would seem less important than that which focuses on the costs and outcomes of care. Further, to conduct research on the latter will require the implementation of an on-line data base containing the essential elements of nursing practice.

ACKNOWLEDGMENT

The authors gratefully acknowledge the assistance of Miaofen Yen in searching and retrieving the literature.

REFERENCES

Abdellah, F. G., & Levine, E. (1965). *Better patient care through nursing research.* New York: Macmillan.

Abdellah, F. G., & Levine, E. (1979). *Better patient care through nursing research* (2nd ed.). New York: Macmillan.

Albrecht, M. N. (1991). Home health care: Reliability and validity testing of a patient-classification instrument. *Public Health Nursing, 8,* 124–131.

Allen, C., Easley, C., & Stofrjell, J. (1986). Cost management through caseload/workload analysis. In F. Shaffer (Ed.) *Patients and purse strings* (pp. 331–346). New York: National League for Nursing.

Ambutas, S. (1987). Evaluating a patient classification system. *DCCN: Dimensions of Critical Care Nursing, 6*(6), 364–367.

Ambutas, S. (1988). A comparison of two patient classification systems for an MICU. *Nursing Management, 19*(9), 64A-C, 64F, 64H.

Arenth, L. M. (1985). The development and validation of an Oncology Patient Classification System. *Oncology Nursing Forum, 12,* 17–22.

Aydelotte, M. K. (1973). *Nursing staffing methodology: A review and critique of selected literature.* (DHEW Pub. No. NIH 73–433). Washington, DC: U.S. Government Printing Office.

Baar, A., Moores, B., & Rhys-Hearn, C. (1973). A review of the various methods of measuring the dependency of patients on nursing staff. *International Journal of Nursing Studies, 10,* 195–203.

Ballard, S., & McNamara, R. (1983). Quantifying nursing needs in home health care. *Nursing Research, 32,* 236–241.

Bay, K. S., Leatt, P., & Stinson, S. M. (1983). Cross-validation of a patient classification procedure: An application of the U method. *Medical Care, 21,* 31–47.

Bigbee, J. L., Collins, J., & Deeds, K. (1992). Patient classification systems: A new approach to computing reliability. *Applied Nursing Research, 5,* 32–37.

Boondas, J. (1991). Nursing home resident assessment classification and focused care. *Nursing & Health Care, 12*, 308–312.

Buchan, I. M. (1979). *Nurse staffing methodology in Canada.* Ottawa: Canadian Nurses' Association.

Burger, J., & Schmitt, P. (1982). Patient classification index documents staffing needs. *Critical Care Nurse, 2*(5), 33–35.

Campbell, M. L. (1988). Accounting for care: A framework for analyzing change in Canadian nursing. In R. White (Ed.), *Political Issues in Nursing: Past, Present and Future* (Vol. 3, pp. 45–70). New York: Wiley.

Canadian Nurses' Association. (1966). *Report on the project for the evaluation of the quality of nursing service.* Ottawa: Author.

Cavaiola, J. H. (1975). *A unified approach to patient classification and nurse staffing for long-term care.* Unpublished doctoral dissertation. The Johns Hopkins University, Baltimore.

Cavaiola, L. J., & Young, J. P. (1980). An integrated system for patient assessment and classification and nurse staff allocation for long term care facilities. *Health Services Research, 15*, 281–306.

Charbonneau, C., Ostrowski, C., Poehner, E. T., Lindsay, P., Panniers, T. L., Houghton, P., & Albright, J. (1988). Validity and reliability issues in alternative patient classification systems. *Medical Care, 26*, 800–813.

Churness, V. H., Kleffel, D., & Onodera, M. (1991). Home health patient classification system. *Home Healthcare Nurse, 9*(2), 14–22.

Cohen, S. M., Arnold, L., Brown, L., & Brooten, D. (1991). Taxonomic classification of transitional follow-up care nursing interventions with low birthweight infants. *Clinical Nurse Specialist, 5*, 31–36.

Connor, R. J. (1960). *A hospital inpatient classification system.* Unpublished doctoral dissertation, The Johns Hopkins University, Baltimore.

Connor, R. J. (1961a). Hospital work sampling with associated measures of production. *Journal of Industrial Engineering, 13*, 105–107.

Connor, R. J. (1961b). A work sampling study of variations in nursing workload. *Hospitals, 35*(9), 40–41.

Connor, R. J., Flagle, C. D., Hseih, R. K. C., Preston, R. A., & Singer, S. (1961). Effective use of nursing resources: A research report. *Hospitals, 35*(5), 30–39.

Cromwell, J., & Harrow, B. (1985). *Summary and critique of patient classification systems.* Contract No. T-31415512. Washington, DC: Health Economics Research.

Cullen, D. J., Civetta, J. M., Briggs, B. A., & Ferrara, L. C. (1974). Therapeutic intervention scoring system: A method for quantitative comparison of patient care. *Critical Care Medicine, 2*(2), 57–60.

Daubert, E. A. (1979). Patient classification system and outcome criteria. *Nursing Outlook, 27*, 450–454.

DeGroot, H. A. (1989). Patient classification system evaluation, Part I: Essential system elements. *Journal of Nursing Administration, 19*(6), 30–35.

Densen, P. M., & Jones, E. W. (1976). The patient classification for long-term care developed by four research groups in the United States. *Medical Care, 14*(Suppl. 5), 126–133.

Donnelly, L. J. (1981). Patient classification: An effective management tool. *Nursing Management, 12*(11), 42–43.

Edwardson, S., Bahr, J., & Serote, M. (1990). Patient classification and management information systems as adjuncts to patient care delivery. In B. B. Mayer, M. J.

Madden, & E. Lawrenz (Eds.), *Patient care delivery models* (pp. 293–313). Rockville, MD: Aspen.

Edwardson, S. R., & Giovannetti, P. B. (1987). A review of cost-accounting methods for nursing services. *Nursing Economics, 5,* 107–117.

Edwardson, S. R., & Nardone, P. (1990). The dependency at discharge instrument as a measure of resource use in home care. *Public Health Nursing, 7,* 138–144.

Ehrman, M. L. (1987). Using a factored patient classification system in Psychiatry. *Nursing Management, 18*(5), 48–50, 53.

Eklof, M., & Qu, W. (1986). Validating a psychiatric patient classification system. *Journal of Nursing Administration, 16*(5), 10–17.

Fetter, R. B., Averill, F. R., Lichtenstein, J. L., & Freeman, J. L. (1984). Ambulatory visit groups: A framework for measuring productivity in ambulatory care. *Health Services Research, 19,* 415–437.

Flowerdew, A. D. J., & Malin, P. W. (1963). Systematic activity sampling. *Journal of Industrial Engineering, 15,* 201–207.

Fries, B. E., & Cooney, L. M. (1985). Resource utilization groups: A patient classification system. *Medical Care, 23,* 110–122.

Genovich-Richards, J., & Tracy, R. L. (1984). An assessment process for nursing staff patterns in ambulatory care. *Journal of Ambulatory Care Management, 7*(2), 69–79.

Giovannetti, P. (1978). *Patient classification systems in nursing: A description and analysis.* (DHEW Pub. No. HRA 78/22). Washington, DC: U.S. Government Printing Office.

Giovannetti, P. (1984). Staffing methods—Implications for quality. In L. Willis & P. Lindwood (Eds.), *Measuring the quality of nursing care* (pp. 123–150). London: Churchill Livingstone.

Giovannetti, P., & Johnson, J. M. (1990). A new generation patient classification system. *Journal of Nursing Administration, 20*(5), 33–40.

Gorham, W. A. (1962). Staff nursing behaviors contributing to patient care and improvement. *Nursing Research, 11,* 68–79.

Haas, S. A. (1988). Patient classification systems: A self-fulfilling prophecy... instruments can limit the scope of nursing. *Nursing Management, 19*(5), 56–58, 60–62.

Hagerty, B. K., Chang, R. S., & Spengler, C. D. (1985). Work sampling: Analyzing nursing staff productivity. *Journal of Nursing Administration, 15*(9), 9–14.

Halloran, E. J. (1985). Nursing workload, medical diagnosis related groups, and nursing diagnoses. *Research in Nursing & Health, 8,* 421–433.

Hanson, R. L. (1979). Issues and methodological problems in nurse staffing research. *Communicating Nursing Research, 12,* 51–56.

Harris, M. D., Santoferraro, C., & Silva, S. (1985). A patient classification system in home health care. *Nursing Economics, 3,* 276–282.

Hastings, C. E. (1987). Classification issues in ambulatory care nursing: Developing a staffing model based on workload analysis. *Journal of Ambulatory Care Management, 10*(3), 50–64.

Hastings, C., & Muir-Nash, J. (1989). Validation of a taxonomy of ambulatory nursing practice. *Nursing Economics, 7,* 142–149.

Hays, B. (1992). Nursing care requirements and resource consumption in home health care. *Nursing Research, 41,* 138–143.

Helberg, J. L. (1989). Reliability of the nursing classification index for home healthcare. *Nursing Management, 20*(3), 48–56.

Hoffman, F., & Wakefield, D. S. (1986). Ambulatory care patient classification. *Journal of Nursing Administration, 16*(4), 23–30.

Hogan, A. J., & Smith, D. W. (1987). Patient classification and resource allocation in Veterans Administration nursing home. *Advances in Nursing Science, 9*(3), 56–71.

Hsiao, W. C., Braun, P., Yntema, D., & Becker, E. R. (1988). Estimating physicians' work for a resource-based relative-value scale. *New England Journal of Medicine, 319,* 835–841.

Jennings, B. M., Rea, R. E., Antopol, B. B., & Carty, J. L. (1989). Selecting, implementing, and evaluating patient classification systems: A measure of productivity. *Nursing Administration Quarterly, 14*(1), 24–35.

Johnson, J. M. (1989). Quantifying an ambulatory care patient classification instrument. *Journal of Nursing Administration, 19*(11), 36–42.

Johnson, K. (1984). A practical approach to patient classification. *Nursing Management, 15*(6), 39–41, 44, 46.

Jones, K. R. (1984). Severity of illness measures: Issues and options. *Nursing Economics, 2,* 312–317.

Joseph, A. C. (1990). Ambulatory care: An objective assessment. *Journal of Nursing Administration, 20*(2), 27–33.

Karshmer, J. F. (1991). Expert nursing diagnoses. The link between nursing care plans and patient classification systems. *Journal of Nursing Administration, 21*(1), 31–39.

Katz, S., Hedrick, S. C., & Henderson, N. S. (1979). The measurement of long-term care needs and impact. *Health and Medical Care Services Review, 2*(1), 1–21.

Keene, R., & Cullen, D. J. (1983). Therapeutic intervention scoring system: Update 1983. *Critical Care Medicine, 11*(1), 1–3.

Lampe, S. (1987). Costing hospital nursing services: A review of the literature (DHHS Pub. [HRSA] HRP-0907983). Springfield, VA: National Technical Information Services.

Leatt, P., Bay, K. S., & Stinson, S. M. (1981). An instrument for assessing and classifying patients by type of care. *Nursing Research, 30,* 145–150.

Lewis, E. N. (1989). *Manual of patient classification: Systems and techniques for practical application.* Rockville, MD: Aspen.

Lindner, C. A. (1989). Work measurement and nursing time standards. *Nursing Management, 20*(10), 44–46, 48–49.

Martin, K. (1982). A client classification system adaptable for computerization. *Nursing Outlook, 30,* 515–517.

Maynard, H. B. (1971). *Industrial engineering handbook.* New York: McGraw-Hill.

McCloskey, J. C., Gardner, D. L., & Johnson, M. R. (1987). Costing out nursing services: An annotated bibliography. *Nursing Economics, 5,* 245–253.

McKenzie, D. A. (1991). A proposed prototype for identifying and correcting sources of measurement error in classification systems. *Medical Care, 29,* 521–530.

Miller, P. L., & Folse, G. H. (1989). Patient classification and staffing in ambulatory care. *Nursing Management, 20*(8), 29–31.

Mitty, E. (1987). Prospective payment and long-term care: Linking payments to resource use. *Nursing & Health Care, 8*(1), 15–21.

Morath, J., Fleischmann, R., & Boggs, G. (1989). A missing consideration: The psychiatric patient classification for scheduling-staffing systems. *Perspectives in Psychiatric Care, 25*(3/4), 40–47.

National League for Nursing Education. (1937). *A study of nursing services in fifty selected hospitals.* New York: Author.

National League of Nursing Education. (1948). *A study of nursing service in one children's and twenty-one general hospitals.* New York: Author.

National League for Nursing Education. (1949). Criteria for assignment of the nursing aid. *American Journal of Nursing, 49,* 311–14.

Niemeier, D. F., & Reed, G. B. (1985). A monitoring system for patient classification in critical care. *DCCN: Dimensions in Critical Care Nursing, 4,* 110–118.

O'Brien-Pallas, L. L. (1987). *Analysis of variation in nursing workload associated with patient's medical and nursing diagnosis and patient classification method.* Unpublished doctoral dissertation, University of Toronto, Toronto, Ontario, Canada.

O'Brien-Pallas, L., & Cockerill, R. (1989). *A study of nursing workload measures.* (Final Report NHW/HSP 285-03524). Ottawa, Ontario, Canada: Health and Welfare Canada.

O'Brien-Pallas, L., Cockerill, R., & Leatt, P. (1991). *A comparison of the workload estimated by five patient classification systems in nursing.* (Final Report No. 6606-3706-57). Ottawa, Ontario, Canada: Health and Welfare Canada.

Pardue, S. F., & Dick, C. T. (1986). Patient classification: Illness acuity and nursing care needs. *Journal of Psychosocial Nursing and Mental Health Services, 24*(12), 23–30.

Parrinello, K., Brenner, P. S., & Vallone, B. (1988). Refining and testing a nursing patient classification instrument in ambulatory care. *Nursing Administration Quarterly, 13*(1), 54–65.

Peters, D. A. (1987). *Development and testing of a community health nursing intensity rating scale for patient classification.* Doctoral Dissertation. University of Pennsylvania, Philadelphia, PA. (0175)

Peters, D. A. (1988). Development of a community health intensity rating scale. *Nursing Research, 37,* 202–207.

Phillips, C. Y., Castorr, A., Prescott, P. A., & Soeken, K. (1992). Nursing intensity: Going beyond patient classification. *Journal of Nursing Administration, 22*(4), 46–52.

Reitz, J. A. (1985a). Toward a comprehensive nursing intensity index: Part I Development. *Nursing Management, 16*(8), 21–24, 26, 28–30.

Reitz, J. A. (1985b). Toward a comprehensive nursing intensity index: Part II Testing. *Nursing Management, 16*(9), 31–32, 34, 36–40, 42.

Ringerman, E. S., & Luz, S. (1990). A psychiatric patient classification system. *Nursing Management, 21*(10), 66–71.

Roehrl, P. K. (1979). Patient classification: A pilot test. *Supervisor Nurse, 10*(3), 21–22, 25–27.

Rookes, P. J. (1982). How many health visitors? *Nursing Times, 78,* 2043–2045.

Saba, V. K., O'Hare, P. A., Zuckerman, E. A., Boondas, J. Levine, E., & Oatway, D. M. (1991). Nursing intervention taxonomy for home health care. *Nursing and Health Care, 12,* 296–299.

Schroeder, R. E., Rhodes, A. M., & Shields, R. E. (1984). Nurse acuity systems: CASH vs. GRASP. *Nursing Forum, 21,* 72–77.

Schroder, P. J., Washington, W. P., Deering, C. D., & Coyne, L. (1986). Testing validity and reliability in a psychiatric patient classification system. *Nursing Management, 17,* 49–50, 52, 54.

Semradek, J., Giovannetti, P., Hornbrook, M., McKenzie, D., Will, S., Buchan, J., Capuzzi, C., Brennan, K., Jahn, J., & Lieber, D. (1988). *Alberta Patient Classification System for Long Term Care Facilities—Final Report.* Edmonton, Alberta, Canada. Alberta Hospitals and Medical Care.

Shade, J. G., & Austin, J. K. (1992). Quantifying ambulatory care activities by time and complexity. *Nursing Economics, 1,* 183–192.

Simmons, D. A. (1980).*A classification scheme for client problems in community health nursing.* (DHHS Publication No. HRA 80-16). Washington, DC: U.S. Government Printing Office.

Soeken, K. L., & Prescott, P. A. (1986). Issues in the use of Kappa to estimate reliability. *Medical Care, 24,* 733–741.

Soeken, K. L., & Prescott, P. A. (1991). Patient intensity for nursing index: The measurement model. *Research in Nursing & Health, 14,* 297–304.

Sovie, M. D. (1988). Variable costs of nursing care in hospitals. In J. J. Fitzpatrick, R. L. Taunton, & J. Q. Benoliel (Eds.), *Annual Review of Nursing Research,* (Volume 6, pp. 13–150). New York: Springer Publishing Co.

Storch, J. L., & Stinson, S. M. (1988). Concepts of depressionalization with applications to nursing. In R. White (Ed.), *Political Issues in Nursing: Past, Present and Future* (vol. 3, pp. 33–44). Toronto: Wiley.

Thibault, C. (1990). *Workload measurement in nursing.* Montreal: Quebec Hospital Association.

Thomas, D. M., & Moses, W. A. (1986). Psychiatric nurses develop their own workload measurement system. *Canadian Journal of Psychiatric Nursing, 27,* 8–12.

Trivedi, V. M. (1979). Nursing judgment in selection of patient classification variables. *Research in Nursing and Health, 2,* 109–118.

Trivedi, V. M. (1982). Measurement of task delegations among nurses by nominal group process analysis. *Medical Care, 20,* 154–164.

United States Department of Health, Education, and Welfare (1978).*Methods for studying nurse staffing in a patient unit: A manual to aid hospitals in making use of personnel.* (DHEW Publication No. HRA 78–3). Hyattsville, MD: Dept. of Health, Education, and Welfare, Public Health Service, Health Resources Administration, Bureau of Health Manpower, Division of Nursing.

Verran, J.A. (1981). Delineation of ambulatory care nursing practice.*Journal of Ambulatory Care Management, 4,* 1–13.

Verran, J. A. (1986a). Patient classification in ambulatory care. *Nursing Economics, 4,* 247–251.

Verran, J. A. (1986b). Testing a classification instrument for the ambulatory care setting. *Research in Nursing & Health, 9,* 279–287.

Whitney, J. D., & Killien, M. G. (1987). Establishing predictive validity of a patient classification system. *Nursing Management, 18*(5), 80–82, 84–86.

Williams, M. A., & Murphy, L. N. (1979). Subjective and objective measures of staffing adequacy. *Journal of Nursing Administration, 9*(11), 21–29.

Wilson-Barnett, J. (1978).*A review of patient-nurse dependency studies.* Unpublished manuscript, England.

Wolfe, H., & Young, J. P. (1965a). Staffing the nursing unit, Part I: Controlled variable staffing. *Nursing Research, 14,* 236–243.

Wolfe, H., & Young, J. P. (1965b). Staffing the nursing unit, Part II: The multiple assignment technique. *Nursing Research, 14,* 299–303.

Young, J. P., Giovannetti, P., Lewison, D., & Thoms, M. L. (1981). *Factors affecting nurse staffing in acute care hospitals: A review and critique of the literature.* (DHEW Pub. No. HRA 81–10). Hyattsville, MD: Division of Nursing.

Chapter 6

Dying Well: Symptom Control Within Hospice Care

INGE B. CORLESS
MGH INSTITUTE OF HEALTH PROFESSIONS

CONTENTS

Practitioners in hospice nursing perceive the hospice movement as an opportunity to address the physical, psychological, social, and spiritual concerns and needs of the client and his or her family so that an individual may die well.

Petrosino (1986a) directed attention to the array of elements comprising hospice nursing including symptom control and management, individualization of care, availability of the nurse, patient–family control, anticipatory care, rapid, effective nursing involvement, and interdisciplinary interactions.

Hospice as a Political Movement

The hospice tradition of exquisite attention to the physical manifestations of terminal illness emanated from Dame Cecily Saunders, the founder of St. Christopher's Hospice in Sydenham, England. Saunders and her colleagues, attempting to demonstrate the validity of this approach, embarked on a series of studies of symptom control beginning wlth determining the efficacy of various pain-relieving modalities (Saunders, 1967; Twycross, 1974, 1977, & 1983). These studies and those by Melzack, Ofeish, and Mount (1976) and Mount, Ajemian, and Scott (1976) contributed to legitimizing palliative care as an approach to care of the terminally ill in Britain.

In the United States, hospice has been primarily a social movement rather than a new medical/health care specialty attempting to legitimate itself with the requisite research-based scientific foundation (Wald, Foster, & Wald, 1980). The charismatic elements of this "happy death" movement sought to develop programs of support enabling persons to die as they would wish. Hospice provided the "something" when "nothing more could be done" (Corless, 1983a). Hospice is thus a place, a philosophy of care, and a program of activities focused on symptom management. This triadic definition creates complexity that was evident in reviewing the studies. Some studies simply used the place, others focused on death and dying as a topic, and still others were on symptom management.

Although accepting the credo of attention to the physical, psychological, social, and spiritual, hospice care providers in the United States were limited by nonreimbursement for inpatient "dying." Further, outpatient visits were reimbursed for skilled nursing on a per visit basis, no matter the length of the visit. The need for new funding mechanisms led to political activism (Torrens, 1986). Hospice activists responded to the goal of the Health Care Financing Administration to cut costs by identifying the potential cost savings to be achieved through hospice programs (Corless, 1984, 1985). The legislation that finally was signed into law was less than ideal but it was at least a beginning (Corless, 1984, 1985).

This legislation was passed while the Health Care Financing Administration was engaged in research to determine whether hospice as an intervention was significantly different from traditional care with regard to such factors as cost, satisfaction with care, symptom control, place of death, and quality of life (Greer et al., 1986, 1987). The emphasis on hospice as an intervention and on interdisciplinary care obscured the role of discrete professions and redirected efforts from individual symptom-related interventions to the global intervention of the hospice itself. This may have contributed to the relative paucity of research on symptom control in hospice nursing.

There were studies done in hospice settings but these projects seemed to focus more on far-advanced diseases rather than symptom management. These studies were primarily about the final stages of disease course in hematological and oncological diseases and therapies. So in reality the fact that they took place in hospice settings was tangential. Selected examples of such studies will be reviewed in this chapter for completeness, but they are not hospice studies in the true sense of the term.

Context of Hospice Literature

Hospice literature occurs in the context of the larger scholarly concerns with death and dying, the scientific/medical concerns of oncology and hematology, and to a lesser extent, the nascent developments in psychoneuroimmunology. The death and dying literature is replete with studies of cultural differences in various death-related practices, developmental differences, as well as phenomena such as suicide, grief, mourning, and bereavement (see Petrosino, 1988, *The Hospice Journal*, Death Studies, Omega). Studies on the concepts of death anxiety and fears among health care workers have been expanded to include studies of burnout in the professional literature (Bram & Katz, 1989; Denton & Wisenbaker, 1977; Hopping, 1977; Lyall, Vachon, & Rogers, 1980; Mallet, Price, Jurs, & Slenker, 1991; Martin, 1981–83; Mor & Laliberte, 1984).

The oncology/hematology literature contains descriptions and evolutions of new technologies, pharmaceuticals and control of drug side effects and other treatment effects. The interest in control of side effects meshes well with the goal in hospice of symptom control (Levy, 1987–88; Wickham, 1989).

Psychoneuroimmunology is helpful not only to discussions of pain but also psychosocial concerns such as the impact of social support on breast cancer survival (Spiegel, Bloom, Kraemer, & Gottheil, 1989). Studies of widowhood and depressed immune system post-bereavement also fit into this tradition (Bartrop, Lazarus, Luckhurst, Kiloh, & Penny, 1977; Schleifer, Keller, Camerino, Thornton, & Stein, 1983).

Symptom Control

Symptom control, also called palliative or supportive care by the medical establishment, is concerned primarily with controlling physical and physical-related symptoms such as pain, nausea, anorexia, diarrhea, dyspnea, decubitus ulcers, anxiety, and confusion-restlessness. Depression is the only psychological phenomenon mentioned as a symptom by Mount (1978) and Geltman and Paige (1983). Although not included in his list of symptoms, Mount (1978) discussed mental distress and the fears of the dying. Moseley (1985) noted anxiety and fear in addition to depression, fatigue, pain, nausea and vomiting, elimination, odor control, nutrition and hydration, breathing, and personal care needs.

Benedict (1990) distinguished between patient-centered and provider-centered research. Symptom control falls within the domain of patient-centered research. Provider-centered research is that which concerns professionals, volunteers, and programs. Research on hospice nurses' death anxiety, and burnout and its prevention, falls within this classification and is beyond the scope of this review. The question of what is effective hospice nursing, however, is both provider-related and patient-related since it addresses questions about the effectiveness of hospice nursing as viewed by the recipient.

Two methodological comments are in order. Hospice nursing as an intervention will be construed as encompassing nursing behavior as an intervention. Symptom control is only one of the repertoire of behaviors comprising nursing. Second, symptom control, which is largely physical and caregiver defined, will be considered to also include patient/family needs as defined by those individuals. Although this enlarges the focus of this review, it reflects the direction of research in the hospice literature.

THE SEARCH PROCESS

The search strategy employed was to cast a wide net using several terms, including symptom(s), nursing, hospice, care, palliative care, terminal illness, symptom control, and pathophysiology.

Only English-language articles were examined. Dissertation abstracts provided names for author searches. Case studies, essays, and editorials on symptom control and hospice nursing were not included. MEDLINE, AIDSline, Health Plan, and Cumulative Index of Nursing and Allied Health Literature (CINAHL) systems were used in the search.

A MEDLINE search was conducted for the years 1986 through August 1992; of 83 articles found, six were relevant. Health Plan was searched from 1981 through May 1992 and provided one article beyond the six from MEDLINE. AIDSline is a newly available database, focused on acquired immune deficiency syndrome (AIDS). The search yielded no relevant studies.

CINAHL's 1983 subject heading list included hospice care; hospice nursing was added in 1987. Four articles were identified using the combined terms hospice, symptoms, and research. Although none strictly speaking met the selection criteria, the paper by Lindley-Davis (1991) merits discussion. *Death Studies* and the *Hospice Journal* were examined starting with volume 8 for *Death Studies* and volume 1 for the *Hospice Journal*. Articles meeting the criteria were included for discussion in the results section.

SYMPTOM PREVALENCE

Symptom control has received only limited attention from researchers concerned with hospice nursing practice. In addition to the symptoms described by Geltman and Paige (1983), Moseley (1985), and Mount (1978) what does the research literature indicate are the symptoms in need of control? In the National Hospice Study on end stage cancer, the following symptoms were commonly reported by patients: "pain 60%, dyspnea 64%, fever 35%, nausea or vomiting 44%, constipation 52%, diarrhea 27%, weight loss 84%, and anorexia 90%. . ." (Wachtel, Allen-Masterson, Reuben, Goldberg, & Mor, 1988). The authors also noted that although only 12% of the participants experienced complete mental incapacitation, a larger segment of the patient population perceived a decrease in their ability to function and their quality of life. The epidemiology of symptoms that comprised part of the National Hospice Study suggested both the traditional domain of symptom control and one with a wider purview, namely that of functional status and quality of life.

The National Hospice Study collected data examining symptoms 4 to 6 weeks predeath and 1 day to 2 weeks predeath. However, these two points in time need additional data points if a more refined understanding of the trajectory of symptoms is to be achieved.

In a retrospective analysis of the charts of 11 deceased clients, Lindley-Davis (1991) found the following objective and subjective phenomena: anorexia 82%; *absence* of pain 55%; nausea/vomiting 36%; apical pulse greater than 100 beats/minute 91%; respirations shallow, labored, and/or periods of apnea 73%; withdrawal defined as repeated periods of nonverbalization 73%; secretions, coughing, congestion, and adventitious lung sounds 64%; decreased mental status 64%; decreased urinary output 64%; restlessness 55%; bowel—hypoactive or incontinence 45%; decreased blood pressure 36%; rectal temperature greater than 99.6 degrees F 36%; skin temperature—cool to touch 36%, skin color—pale, mottled, cyanotic 36%; edema 27%; and diaphoresis 9%. These symptoms encompass what might be termed "active dying." In these retrospective reviews authors did not examine the occurrence of symptoms from a trajectory perspective. The retrospective nature of the Lindley-Davis (1991) analysis depends on the completeness of the charting, and the length of time in the hospice program may underestimate the prevalence of these symptoms and others. The small number ($n = 11$) of charts reviewed may result in under- or over-estimation in extrapolating to a larger population.

SYMPTOM PREVALENCE AND UTILIZATION OF INPATIENT CARE

What is the relationship between symptom prevalence and the utilization of inpatient care? Hays (1986) explored the question of "the relationships among patient symptoms, family anxiety and fatigue, the patterns of hospice service utilization" and ultimately which patients required inpatient care by examining 50 charts each of persons who did and did not receive inpatient care for symptoms during the last 10 days of life. The most prevalent symptoms were pain, nausea/vomiting, respiratory distress, elimination problems, nutritional deficit, and mental status deficit (Hays, 1986). Other problems mentioned included skin problems, body image changes, immobility, fatigue, insomnia, mood changes, and anxiety. More symptoms and more combinations of symptoms indicated patients were at risk for institutionalization (Hays, 1986). It was not possible to isolate the contribution of nursing care in this study.

The severity of nursing care problems and the availability of support at home was found to distinguish those who use inpatient or home hospice care (Mor, Wachtel, & Kidder, 1985). In particular, use of intravenous therapy and bowel and bladder dependence were variables that distinguished those who were cared for at home or in an institution. Although intravenous therapy may no longer be a differentiating factor given the growth of outpatient and at-home infusion therapy, it is likely that bowel and bladder dependence is still a major concern in providing care in the home. It is important to note that no hospice nursing studies of interventions addressing incontinence were located. In addition to severity of nursing care problems, the availability of supportive care at home was identified by multivariate logistic regression to distinguish those persons admitted to a hospital-based program of care. Those individuals without the necessary informal caregiver support may have elected hospital-based hospices to give them the ongoing support they needed. It seems germane to note that the availability of a range of supportive hospice services also may make it possible for those in a resource-poor environment to remain at home.

RESEARCH ON SYMPTOM CONTROL

The symptoms discussed in this section are anorexia, pressure ulcers, pain, delirium, and dyspnea. The reader will note the absence of a number of important symptoms affecting the dying person; possible reasons for the lack of research on certain symptoms will be addressed.

Anorexia

In a study of anorexia, Holden (1991) met with 14 patient-caregiver pairs to investigate, . . . , via semistructured interviews the views and responses of these participants to loss of appetite. Female caregivers were more concerned about loss of appetite than were males. Patients viewed anorexia as less significant than some other problems such as pain, breathing problems, weakness, fear of death, and were more likely to focus on what had been consumed. Holden noted that changes in dietary patterns occurred in all but one of the caregivers as well. Although not an intervention study, the data provided an understanding of the impact of loss of appetite to the patient-caregiver dyad and offered useful basic information to the development of interventions to assist the caregiver.

Pressure Ulcers

In a comparative analysis of two methods of predicting the prevalence and incidence of pressure ulcer occurrence, Hanson et al. (1991) examined prospective and retrospective approaches. Data were collected in two phases using the Braden Scale for Predicting Pressure Ulcer Risk (Bergstrom, Braden, Lagozza, & Hoffman, 1982), and a skin assessment tool based on Shea's staging of a pressure ulcer adapted by the National Pressure Ulcer Advisory Panel in 1989 (Shea, 1989; National Pressure Advisory Panel, 1989). In phase I, one of eight hospice patients receiving care was found to have stage two ulcers, a prevalence rate of 13%. In the phase-II prospective study the incidence of pressure ulcers in 19 hospice patients over a 4-week period was zero, although Braden scores indicated significant risk. The retrospective risk over 9 months for 61 other patients was 13%, that is, eight persons developed 13 pressure ulcers. All of these individuals used hospital beds and were cared for at home. Urinary continence was a factor in two of these eight persons and incontinence of the bowel also was noted in two of the eight persons. It is not clear whether the same persons experienced incontinence of both bladder and bowel. The results suggest that when high-risk individuals are identified, pressure sores can be prevented. The results also may be a reflection of the methodology in that prospective patients were assessed for the first 4 weeks after admission, which is not the time of greatest risk. Hanson et al. (1991) found that the majority of pressure ulcers developed within 2 weeks of death. Further research is required to specify the most critical variables for individuals not otherwise identified as at risk. Hanson and colleagues

(1991), however, provided a foundation by identifying factors that may lead to pressure ulcer development.

Effective treatment of pressure sores has been as important a topic for clinicians as has the prevention of their development. The use of Omiderm (Omikron Scientific Ltd., Rehoret, Israel), a polyurethene-based dressing, was investigated with the 22 first- and second-degree pressure sores of 16 hospice patients (Goren, 1989). Sores with black discoloration or extension into the muscle tissue were not included. Complete healing occurred in 45% of the sores, partial healing in 27% of the pressure sores, and no change was the finding in the remaining 27% of the sores. The researcher did not compare the use of Omiderm with any other method so the relative efficacy of Omiderm was not addressed. Goren (1989) did note the need for exploring the use of Omiderm with more invasive pressure sores.

Pain

Pain has been identified as an accompaniment to far-advanced disease for many persons in various settings (Dobratz, Burns, & Oden, 1989; Morris et al., 1986). It is one of the symptoms wherein the team approach is taken. Saunders (1967) used the term "total pain" to encompass the physical, psychological, spiritual, and social components of pain in advanced cancer. Hospice nurses have incorporated the findings of other colleagues both in hospice and in oncology in their care of patients, but have not taken a leadership role in generating new knowledge on this topic.

The efficacy of discrete pain modalities as well as the relationship of pain to quality of life have been the foci for research. In a clinical trial of short-acting versus controlled-release analgesia, Ferrell, Wisdom, Wenzl, and Brown (1989) demonstrated the validity of one of the main tenets of hospice care, namely that round-the-clock medication is more efficacious than as-needed (prn) dispensing. This study was unique in that it is one of few studies conducted as a randomized clinical trial. Another unique feature was that quality of life was measured as a form of validation of the success of pain relief. The importance of quality of life measurements in pain relief is that data on pain relief may not capture the undesired side effects accompanying certain types and dosages of analgesics.

An extension of this research to the route of medication examined controlled release medication MS Contin (Purdue Frederick Company, Norwalk, CT) by rectal suppository as an alternative to the oral route (Maloney, Kesner, Klein, & Bockenstette, 1989). The study used chart review of 39 terminally ill persons to discover whether pain relief was maintained in these patients with the change in delivery system. Although the study validated the efficacy of rectal administration subsequent to oral administration, it was not a randomized controlled trial but rather a case study of change in route of administration as a response to persistent side effects with oral administration. Accuracy of results was dependent on the adequacy of documentation, an issue not addressed by the researchers. Nonetheless, studies such as this can provide a foundation for future studies on the impact of route of administration.

The adequacy of pain management in hospice home care has been examined by two groups of researchers. In a retrospective study of pain in 30 hospice home care patients (Dobratz, Wade, Herbst, & Ryndes, 1991), charts were examined for changes in numerical pain intensity ratings and changes in route or scheduling of medications. Twenty of the 30 patients experienced steady escalating pain over the course of their hospice stay. For these individuals 23 changes in route of administration were recorded, most frequently to the rectal route. In addition there were 53 changes in medication dosage and scheduling. The researchers found change of medication route to be associated with an increase in perceived pain. A number of topics were identified for further study including the trajectory of pain, that is, stable, declining or escalating, modalities of pain control, the factors significant for effective pain control at home, and the methodological issues related to pain measurement. This study was limited by the inconsistent use of numerical pain ratings, particularly for those individuals who were not experiencing increasing pain. This was a problem of the data, namely the nursing notes. Although the authors acknowledge that few studies have examined the impact of skilled nursing intervention on control of pain over the course of terminal illness in the home they did not examine nursing intervention (Dobratz et al., 1991). Rather, the researchers examined nursing assessment as a vehicle for exploring pain management.

An earlier investigation of pain management in hospice home care examined such patient variables as age, living arrangements, primary cancer site, and compliance with analgesic regimen (Austin, Cody, Eyres, Hefferin, & Krasnow, 1986). Conducting a 2-year retrospective chart review of patients with a prognosis of 1 year or less and a minimum of 2 weeks of hospice care with at least three home care nurse pain assessments, the investigators located 96 patient records eligible for intensive study. Pain intensity in these patients was rated as mild ($n = 26$), moderate ($n = 30$), or severe ($n = 40$). The researchers did not comment on the finding that all of these patients had some pain. Primary cancer site, notably brain, breast, lymphoma, Hodgkin's, and sarcoma correlated with compliance and pain control. Interestingly, 55.2% of patients experiencing pain were noncompliant for a variety of reasons including a concern about addiction, the wish to delay medication until it was really needed, a concern with maintaining control and avoiding dependency, and using the pain as a reminder that they were still living. The researchers recognized the need for a prospective design with both quantitative and qualitative data so that the nature of the patients' support system and coping methods could be investigated. Once again the focus of this study was not nursing intervention but symptom control related to patient variables as determined by retrospective inspection of pain intensity ratings and other data available in the chart. Furthermore, what is considered hospice home care may in fact be home care contracted by hospice programs. When the latter occurs, the service provided may not be to terminally ill persons and hence, may not incorporate the hospice approach. So mixing in such data would contaminate the results from true hospice programs.

Delirium

A study of the frequency, nature, and possible causes of delirium may have inflated the incidence found (85% in the 13 terminally ill cancer patients studied) given that mild difficulties in one-third of the items on mental status, cognitive function, affect, and behavior were considered indicative of delirium (Massie, Holland, & Glass, 1983). In addition, six patients originally considered terminal were discharged and were not included in the data analysis. The findings apply therefore to terminally ill individuals who died during a given admission.

Nurses were noted by the researchers to have a role in helping to allay anxiety, by providing observation for severely agitated, delusional, or hallucinating patients or through continuity in staffing. The recommendations emanating from the study did not address further examination of iatrogenic occurrences such as the interaction between pain medication dosage and discrete phenomena such as brain metastases and metabolic imbalances, although these phenomena were noted to occur. Considering that this study was conducted at a cancer center, one wonders whether replication in a hospice program using the same method would have produced similar results. Furthermore, this study did not investigate nursing interventions that might be used with individuals experiencing different levels of delirium. The National Hospice Study (Wachtel et al., 1988) found that with the exception of persons with a diagnosis of primary or secondary brain cancer, 33.3% of their participants did not exhibit a decrease in mental awareness within 2 weeks of death. Given that patient comfort and patient–family communication are both hospice goals, and may at times be in conflict, further inquiry into this topic would fit within the purview of hospice nursing.

Dyspnea

In an excellent article, Gift (1990) reviewed the research on dyspnea. The patient populations used most frequently in research on dyspnea are those with chronic obstructive pulmonary diseases (COPD), asthma, and lung cancer and not terminally ill persons. As noted previously, dyspnea is a prominent symptom in the terminally ill and thus an important topic for hospice nursing research (Reuben & Mor, 1985). A number of interventions for dyspnea in the terminally ill were suggested by Carrieri and Janson-Bjerklie (1986), Enck (1989), Geltman and Paige (1983), Gift (1990), and Mount (1978), but outcome studies have not been reported.

Hospice as the Intervention

From the state of the literature, one would assume that the unknowns about symptom control concern application rather than the efficacy of different interventions. This would be a fallacious assumption. The major thrust in hospice research has been to examine the impact of the hospice innovation per se rather than discrete symptom control interventions, with the possible exception of pain control (Corless, 1987–1988). In tandem with the political objectives, the emphasis of hospice care on the psychological, social, and spiritual aspects of the patient and the family has resulted in a broader perspective by hospice nurses as to their mandate.

The impact of death on the survivor, typically widows, is illustrative of the sort of research germane to the broader view of what is meant by hospice nursing. An examination of the differences in survivorship experiences of 60 individuals by participation in a hospice program, place of death, length of enrollment in the hospice program, and length of illness was explored using the Grief Experience Inventory (GEI), a 135 true/false item 17 subscale inventory (Sanders, 1978). Significant differences were found in three of the four hypotheses (Steele, 1990). Only length of time enrolled in hospice care prior to death resulted in nonsignificant differences in the grief experience of the survivors. Discriminant function analysis was used to predict group membership based on a number of variables and did so for at least 70% of the cases in the three hypotheses that were supported. Participants in a hospice program were significantly ($p = 0.002$) different from nonparticipants in atypical responses, guilt, loss of control, depersonalization, optimism/despair, dependency and social desirability, survivors of persons who died in the home were significantly ($p = 0.05$) different on denial, guilt, social isolation, rumination, and death anxiety. Lastly, there were significant ($p = 0.04$) differences in those diagnosed with a terminal illness less than 6 months prior to death and those diagnosed with a terminal illness more than 6 months prior to death. Survivors of those diagnosed less than 6 months prior to death scored higher on dependency, social isolation, anger/hostility, and lower on loss of control. The investigators used discriminant analysis as an adjustment since patients were not randomly assigned to the hospice. Thus, research such as that by Steele (1990) provided support for hospice as a global intervention. It does not suggest which nursing interventions, per se, were helpful as do the studies by Freihofer and Felton (1976), Hull (1989, 1991, 1992), and Skorupka and Bohnet (1982), which will be discussed in the next section.

EXPANDING THE HOSPICE CLIENT TO INCLUDE FAMILY

Congruency of Expectations

Questions such as the similarity in perceptions of the problems and strengths of the hospice client by the client, family caregiver, and nurse are the sort that might well be asked in a variety of settings. One could argue that this sort of study is less about hospice than about how isomorphism of perspective affects satisfaction with care.

The instrument developed in a pilot study by Masters and Shontz (1989), based on the work of Padilla et al. (1983), examined performance, attitudes and affective states, well-being, and support as viewed by client, primary caregiver, and hospice nurse. The 27 instrument items addressed the breadth of hospice concerns. Patients perceived themselves as having more strengths than did nurses who were more aware of the problems. Given the small sample, ($n = 20$) clients, ($n = 20$) caregivers, and ($n = 8$) nurses, the authors refrained from generalizing their finding.

Curtis and Fernsler (1989) asked a similar question of 23 patient-caregiver pairs comparing patient and family caregiver assessments. They used the Quality of Life Index developed by Padilla et al. (1983). The tool included medical cost in addition to questions on symptom control, quality of life, and life satisfaction. Initially used with oncology patients, it seems appropriate for this group and other individuals with chronic illnesses. Curtis and Fernsler noted that responses to the tool are indicative of the openness of communication between patient and caregiver. There were no significant differences in patient and caregiver perspectives of the patient's quality of life other than in the area of pain, where patients reported less pain than did their caregivers. No explanation for this difference was offered. Hospice patients had higher scores on symptom control than did the inpatient oncology patient comparison group in Padilla's (1983) study. The design did not control for diagnosis or stage of disease so should be interpreted with caution.

A number of studies have examined nursing behaviors perceived to be helpful by caregiving families. Skorupka and Bohnet (1982) used a Q-sort methodology with 20 hospice family caregivers over a 4-month period. The researchers examined content validity with the assistance of six nurse experts in the content area. A pilot study with 10 families indicated high test–retest reliability. Hospice caregivers sorted the 75 statements into most helpful and least helpful behaviors. The participants were asked to sort the cards into seven piles by actually desired rather than observed behaviors. Furthermore, the number of cards in the most and least helpful piles were three each, the next category/pile from either extreme contained 9 statements, then 15 statements, with the neutral pile containing 21 statements. Researchers found that nursing behaviors related to the patient's physical and emotional needs were more significant to caregivers than meeting their own needs. The most helpful behavior for the male group was "help me locate special equipment (e.g., a hospital bed) to make the patient more comfortable," and for the female group, "provide the patient with necessary emergency measures if the need arises." The top-ranking behavior for the total group was similar to the female group. The least desired behavior for the total group was "cry with me," for the male group, "be open to talking about spiritual matters with the patient." The least desired behavior was not stated for the female group. Although the authors discussed the limitations of sample size on the generalizability of their findings, they failed to address the influence of gender on the findings for the total group. The participants consisted of 12 females, 5 males, and 3 respondents for whom data on gender was missing; hence, total group findings were heavily influenced by the females.

Family Perceptions of Hospice Care

A retrospective study of the perceptions of a convenience sample of 20 bereaved caregivers on the quality of life of their terminally ill family member builds on the research of Skorupka and Bohnet (McGinnis, 1986). Prior to data collection, the investigator administered a Q-sort ranking of preference for 60 nursing behaviors as a test of content validity to hospice nurses on the state hospice council. There was 100% agreement regarding the content validity of the items. Research participants were asked to rate each behavior on a scale of 1 (most helpful) to 7 (least helpful). Most helpful was "teach me to recognize the signs that death is approaching," "stay with the patient during difficult times," and "answer my questions honestly, openly, and willingly." The three least helpful behaviors were "help me make funeral arrangements," "describe how to keep the patient well groomed," and "plan for me to talk about my feelings with other people facing the same problems." It seems plausible that if this research was repeated at different points in the illness trajectory, different behaviors would be more salient. As McGinnis noted, the nursing behaviors valued most may differ depending on whether the caregiver is receiving services from a home care program or an inpatient care program. Program type, often associated with the quality of social support, also may affect desired nursing behaviors. Contrary to the Skorupka and Bohnet results, McGinnis

(1986) found nursing behaviors that addressed the patient's "physical and psychosocial needs and their own (caregiver) psychosocial needs" nearly equally.

Degner, Gow, and Thompson (1991), in semistructured interviews with 10 nursing educators with expertise in death and dying and 10 palliative care nurses, identified seven critical nursing behaviors in caring for the dying. These included responding during the death scene, providing comfort, responding to anger, enhancing personal growth, responding to colleagues, enhancing the quality of life during dying, and responding to the family. Providing comfort entails efforts to reduce physical discomfort, including symptom control. Burns and Carney (1986) sought to identify the nurse's role by examining patterns of time allocation. Although the study did not specify the content of the role, it identified patterns of interaction both via the telephone and in home visits and the periods of greatest intensity of interaction, namely upon admission and discharge. A similar finding was presented by Corless (1983b).

COPING WITH DYING—STRATEGIES

Understanding the coping strategies used by families in hospice home care is basic to developing effective psychosocial interventions. Hull's longitudinal, qualitative study (1991) of coping by 14 individuals from 10 families contributed to this goal. Using semistructured interviews ($n = 55$) and participant observation, Hull (1991) investigated the nature of caring support as perceived by the 10 caregiving families. Hull (1992) used purposive sampling, but unfortunately, bias was introduced because the busiest families were unable to participate in her study (Hull, 1989). Eight of the 10 refusals were by women over 65 years of age. Interestingly nine out of 10 patients experienced mental status changes including confusion, difficulty communicating, and irritability. Coping with these changes was the most problematic aspect of caring for their relatives. Helpful to the families were 24-hour accessibility to nurses, effective communication, a nonjudgmental attitude, and clinical competence. Symptom control needs to be defined more broadly in a hospice context to include the concerns of caregivers. In contrast with earlier findings, information seeking was not used as a coping strategy. Coping techniques used included obtaining respite in "windows of time," social comparison, cognitive reformulation, avoidance, "taking one day at a time," acceptance and rationalization, and social support (Hull, 1992). Verification by families of transcribed interviews, examination of emergent categories by colleagues and acquaintances who had experienced a family member's death, and analysis of data segments by colleagues to validate interpretations were strengths of this study.

COPING WITH DYING—NEEDS

In a qualitative study of hospice patient and family concerns, Lev (1991) interviewed 10 patients and 24 family members. Most frequently expressed were concerns about health. Communication with the doctor, the meaning of life, discharge disposition, work-related concerns, social support, and emotional responses also were expressed as concerns. As with families with a member in a presumably terminal condition in an acute care facility (O'Brien Abt, 1983), information needs were significant to this group of individuals. Although Lev notes that interventions that promote family member strengths, provide information, and emphasize choice are helpful, she also states that "Allowing patients and families to identify their own needs is more appropriate than assuming that all people want or need to face loss similarly" (Lev, 1991).

SATISFACTION WITH CARE

The concerns and coping abilities of widows were identified by Wegmann (1987) using the F Copes Inventory (McCubbin, Larsen, & Olson, 1982), and Jalowiec Coping Scale (Jalowiec, 1979; Jalowiec, Murphy, & Powers, 1984) with individuals who received hospice home care ($n = 32$) or hospital services ($n = 36$). Wegman (1987) found that the nonhospice group used more "active, take charge" types of behavior in coping, whereas the hospice group used more passive affective behaviors such as drug use, withdrawal, and allowing others to make decisions for them. Interviews with five widows from each group resulted in the stunning finding that only one widow would use hospice again, one was uncertain, and eight women indicated they would not. The women listed stresses, uncertainties, and problems with symptom management during their husbands' last days. These all are areas in which descriptive studies and intervention development and testing are needed.

The degree to which the emotional need satisfaction of the familial caregiver is linked to overall satisfaction is evident in Dawson's study (1991) of three different types of hospice programs and a conventional care program. Hospice home care, wherein the patient remained at home to die, resulted in both the highest overall satisfaction and satisfaction with care received from the nurse. Statistically significant Pearson correlations supported the hypothesis that overall satisfaction is negatively related to unmet basic needs ($r = -0.69$) and positively related to the psychosocial support received from nurses ($r = 0.73$) (Dawson, 1991).

Seale's (1989, 1991) comparison of hospice and conventional care in England found that various aspects of care received by a terminally ill family member from a physician were considered to be excellent by 91% of relatives when in hospice and by 40% of relatives when in the hospital. Nurses and other staff were thought to provide excellent care by 96% of relatives when care was given in hospice and 57% of relatives when care was given in the hospital (Seale, 1991). Respondents also felt that they received more assurance at home from hospice nurses (92%) as compared with district nurses (69%).

Comparisons such as these are useful additions to studies that explore the impact of hospice or palliative care on a group of patients (Walsh, 1990). Historical comparisons with previous care (Godkin, Krant, & Doster, 1983–84) or of palliative care over time (Bruera, MacMillan, Hanson, & MacDonald, 1990) are the early studies that foster the development of an innovation such as hospice but are not as powerful scientifically as those with a contemporaneous control group.

SUMMARY AND RECOMMENDATIONS FOR RESEARCH

Studies of symptom control in hospice nursing may have been unduly restricted by the philosophy of hospice and the political environment in which this health care innovation was developed. The philosophy of hospice care requires a blending of professional roles, thus transforming the multidisciplinary team into an interdisciplinary one. The emphasis on the psychological, social, and spiritual as well as on the physical, the family as well as the patient, during dying, death, and bereavement resulted in a larger sphere of caregiving activity than is the situation in traditional care. Likewise it produced a more complex phenomenon for research than traditional care. Lastly, the political need to prove the value of the hospice approach led to investigations that focused on hospice as an intervention compared with nontraditional approaches to terminal care. Although costs were a primary concern, other outcomes also were investigated. The hospice intervention thus was conceptualized as the totality of hospice care and its impact on a variety of outcomes including satisfaction with care. There was much less attention focused on the outcome of controlling a discrete symptom such as pain. It is not surprising that Degner et al. (1991) observed that the literature "contained a systematic bias toward the assessment phase of the nursing process, as opposed to the intervention phase."

Methodologically, the approaches used primarily included retrospective medical record analysis, case study and its variations, Q-sort techniques, and rarely, randomized controlled trials (RCT). Petrosino (1988) noted that prior to the development of intervention studies, there is the need for good descriptive studies and qualitative research. She stated elsewhere (1986b) "in order to build a scientific base for hospice nursing practice, the range of human responses to terminal illness must be explored and described."

Where does that leave the researcher interested in symptom control in hospice nursing? Clearly with room to make contributions which will have an impact on practice. To begin with, it could be useful to rethink "medical" records so that intake records include a review of symptoms and data useful to the formulation of nursing diagnoses. Such information would provide aggregate data on the occurrence of various symptoms in different populations of patients and the human responses to these symptoms. These records could also serve as the foundation for repeated measurements to assess the efficacy of various interventions. An investigation-guided record system offers the basis for the conduct of retrospective studies and randomized controlled trials. The occurrence of symptoms and responses can be formulated to capture presence and degree of severity. Efficacy of intervention can be measured clinically in terms of reduction in severity and from a research perspective with regard to the desirability of different interventions. Such a database might also provide the information necessary for quality assurance and continuous quality improvement programs. The recent emphasis on outcomes research provides further impetus to as research on effective symptom control.

Given the data which demonstrate that effective symptom control is key to maintaining persons in their homes, further research on the identification of factors that precipitate reinstitutionalization seems paramount. In this regard, approaches to alleviating and/or dealing with incontinence seems another obvious area of inquiry given the observation by Halloran (personal communication, 1992) of the significance of this symptom for nursing home placement.

Pain control is a continuing area of concern to patients, families, and professionals. The efficacy of transdermal patches as contrasted with the standard of care, oral morphine, seems another area in which research would be useful. Transdermal patches may also resolve the problem of provision of narcotics to a terminally ill person when other family members may be pilfering the patient's drugs or the patient is an addict. With the acknowledgment that persons with acquired immune deficiency syndrome (AIDS) should have access to hospice care, a variety of problems have surfaced. Among these are the challenges posed in giving care to terminally ill drug users. Innovations such as transdermal patches may have a significant role to play.

Dementia, or its symptom—confusion—is a particular problem for individuals with end-stage AIDS. Care of the patient at home (or in the hospital) is more difficult in the presence of severe confusion. Research on nursing approaches to the care of persons with dementia and other forms of cognitive impairment could make an important contribution.

Although hospice philosophy supports a low technology/low invasiveness approach to terminal illness care, technology may also be explored with regard to its contribution to quality of life. Such technology includes omaya reservoirs, implantable pumps and tubes, various types of beds, wheelchairs, and other equipment, computers, other communication systems, and robots. Technology may assist individuals who live alone to remain at home for much of the terminal illness. Such technology is not proposed to supplant human contact but to supplement it and to enhance independence and quality of life.

Given the tradeoffs that seem inherent in being terminally ill, an exploration of the patient's values and the impact of this calculus on individualizing care seems long overdue (Corless, 1992). Value-imbued care is theorized to, at the least, result in greater client satisfaction and may enhance symptom control. Research that employs a standardized tool to elicit values as the basis for the intervention of individualization could assure quality of life as perceived by the patient and family caregiver. And although perceived control may be an important intervening variable, the values calculus combined with symptom assessment provides a basis for developing a client-centered program of care.

Quality of life, and not just life itself, are important in care provided under the aegis of a hospice program. Hospice advocates have often spoken of patients "living" until they die. The subtext of living until death is one of quality of life. To save hospice nursing research in symptom control from inane clinical trials, the question of quality of life must always be addressed. The good end of life as well as the good death are fitting questions in framing research on hospice nursing.

Johanson (1991) called for studies of the last 48 hours of life, the effectiveness of previous symptom control, the setting of the death, and the available support whether in home, hospice, or elsewhere. Hull (1990) suggested that the role of the hospice nurse be examined. Dobratz (1990) proposed that hospice nurses engage in the management of physical, psychological, social, and spiritual problems of dying persons and their family members. Dobratz (1990) called this "intensive caring" and included collaborative sharing, continuous knowing, and continuous giving. This conceptualization is analogous to symptom control.

REFERENCES`

Austin, C., Cody, C. P., Eyres, P. J., Hefferin, E. A., & Krasnow, R. W. (1986). Hospice home care pain management—four critical variables. *Cancer Nursing, 9*, 58–65.

Bartrop, R. W., Lazarus, L., Luckhurst, E., Kiloh, L. G., & Penny, R. (1977). Depressed lymphocyte function after bereavement. *The Lancet, 1*, 834–836.

Benedict, S. (1990). Nursing research priorities related to HIV/AIDS. *Oncology Nursing Forum, 17*, 571–573.

Benoliel, J. Q. (1983). Nursing research on death, dying and terminal illness: Development, present state and prospects. In H. H. Werley & J. J. Fitzpatrick (Eds.), *Annual Review of Nursing Research* (Vol. 1, pp. 101–130). New York: Springer Publishing Co.

Bergstrom, N., Braden, R. J., Lagozza, A., & Holman, V. (1987). The Braden Scale for Predicting Pressure Sore Risk. *Nursing Research, 36*, 205–210.

Bloom, J. A., & Flannery, J. (1989). Problems in an AIDS hospice setting [Abstract]. *International Conference on AIDS, 5*, 414 (Abstract no. WBP378).

Bram, P. J., & Katz, L. F. (1989). A study of burnout in nurses working in hospice and hospital oncology settings. *Oncology Nursing Forum, 16*, 555–560.

Brege, J. A. (1985–1986). Terminal care: A bibliography of the medical and nursing literature. *The Hospice Journal, 1*, 55–76.

Bruera, E., MacMillan, K., Hanson, J., & MacDonald, R. N. (1990). Palliative care in a cancer center: Results in 1984 versus 1987. *Journal of Pain and Symptom Management, 5*, 1–5.

Burns, N., & Carney, K. (1986). Patterns of hospice care—the RN role. *The Hospice Journal, 2*, 37–61.

Carrieri, V. K., & Janson-Bjerklie, S. (1986). Strategies patients use to manage the sensation of dyspnea. *Western Journal of Nursing Research, 8*, 284–305.

Corless, I. B. (1983a). The hospice movement in North America. In C. Corr & D. Corr (Eds.), *Hospice care: Principles and practice* (pp. 335–351). New York: Springer Publishing Co.

Corless, I. B. (1983b). Research strikes again or the case of the missing nurse visits. Paper presented at the *National Hospice Organization Annual Meeting*. Minneapolis, MN: November 11.

Corless, I. B. (1984). Hospice: The state of the art. In *Proceedings of the Fourth National Conference on Cancer Nursing*. American Cancer Society, 29–35.

Corless, I. B. (1985). Implications of the new hospice legislation and the accompanying regulations. *Nursing Clinics of North America, 20*, 281–298.

Corless, I. B. (1987–1988). Settings for terminal care. *Omega, 18*, 319–340.

Corless, I. B. (1992). Hospice and hope: An incompatible duo. The *American Journal of Hospice and Palliative Care, 9*, 10–11.

Curtis, A. E., & Fernsler, J. I. (1989). Quality of life of oncology hosice patients: A comparison of patient and primary caregiver reports. *Oncology Nursing Forum, 16*, 49–53.

Dawson, N. J. (1991). Need satisfaction in terminal care settings. *Social Science & Medicine, 32*, 83–87.

Degner, L. G., Gow, C. M., & Thompson, L. A. (1991). Critical nursing behaviors in care for the dying. *Cancer Nursing, 14*, 246–253.

Denton, J. A., & Wisenbaker, V. B. (1977). Death experience and death anxiety among nurses and nursing students. *Nursing Research, 26*, 61–64.

Dobratz, M. C. (1990). Hospice nursing. Present perspectives and future directives. *Cancer Nursing, 13*, 116–122.

Dobratz, M. C., Burns, K. M., & Oden, R. V. (1989). Pain in home hospice patients: An exploratory descriptive study. *The Hospice Journal, 5*, 117–133.

Dobratz, M. C., Wade, R., Herbst, L., & Ryndes, T. (1991). Pain efficacy in home hospice patients—a longitudinal study. *Cancer Nursing, 14*, 20–26.

Enck, R. E. (1989). The management of dyspnea. *American Journal of Hospice Care, 6*, 11–12.

Ferrell, B., Wisdom, C., Wenzl, C., & Brown, J. (1989). Effects of controlled-release morphine on quality of life for cancer pain. *Oncology Nursing Forum, 16*, 521–526.

Freihofer, P., & Felton, G. (1976). Nursing behaviors in bereavement: An exploratory study. *Nursing Research, 25*, 332–337.

Geltman, R. L., & Paige, R. L. (1983). Symptom management in hospice care. *American Journal of Nursing, 83*, 78–85.

Gift, A. G. (1990). Dyspnea. *Nursing Clinics of North America, 25*, 955–965.

Godkin, M. A., Krant, M. J., & Doster, N. J. (1983–1984). The impact of hospice care on families. *International Journal of Psychiatry in Medicine, 13*, 153–165.

Goren, D. (1989). Use of omiderm in treatment of low-degree pressure sores in terminally ill cancer patients. *Cancer Nursing, 12*, 165–169.

Greer, D. S., Mor, V., Morris, J. N., Sherwood, S., Kidder, D., & Birnbaum, H. (1986). An alternative in terminal care: Results of the National Hospice Study. *Journal of Chronic Diseases, 39*, 9–26.

Hanson, D., Langemo, D. K., Olson, B., Hunter, S., Sauvage, T. R., Burt, C., & Cathcart-Silverberg, T. (1991). The prevalence and incidence of pressure ulcers in the hospice setting: Analysis of two methodologies. *American Journal of Hospice and Palliative Care, 8*, 18–22.

Hays, J. C. (1986). Patient symptoms and family coping—predictors of hospice utilization patterns. *Cancer Nursing, 9*, 317–325.

Holden, C. M. (1991). Anorexia in the terminally ill cancer patient: The emotional impact on the patient and the family. *The Hospice Journal, 7*, 73–84.

Hopping, B. L. (1977). Nursing students' attitudes toward death. *Nursing Research, 26*, 443–447.

Hull, M. M. (1989). A family experience: Hospice supported home care of a dying relative. (Doctoral dissertation, University of Rochester), UMI order #PUZ 8912968.

Hull, M. M. (1990). Sources of stress for hospice caregiving families. *The Hospice Journal, 6*, 29–54.

Hull, M. M. (1991). Hospice nurses—caring support for caregiving familes. *Cancer Nursing, 14*, 63–70.

Hull, M. M. (1992). Coping strategies of family caregivers in hospice homecare. *Oncology Nursing Forum, 19*, 1179–1187.

Jalowiec, A. (1979). *Jalowiec Coping Scale*. Chicago: University of Illinois.

Jalowiec, A., Murphy, S., & Powers, M. (1984). Psychometric assessment of the Jalowiec Coping Scale. *Nursing Research, 33*, 157–161.

Kane, R. L., Wales, J., Bernstein, L., Leibowitz, A., & Kaplan, S. (1984). A randomized controlled trial of hospice care. *The Lancet, 1*, 890–894.

Lev, E. L. (1991). Dealing with loss: Concerns of patients and families in a hospice setting. *Clinical Nurse Specialist, 5*, 87–93.

Levy, M. H. (1987–1988). Pain control research in the terminally ill. *Omega, Journal of Death and Dying, 18*, 265–280.

Lindley-Davis, B. (1991). Process of dying: Defining characteristics. *Cancer Nursing, 14*, 328–333.

Lyall, A., Vachon, M., & Rogers, J. (1980). A study of the degree of stress experienced by professionals caring for dying patients. In I. Ajemian & B. M. Mount (Eds.), *R.V.H. manual on palliative/hospice care* (pp. 498–500). New York: Arno Press.

Mahoney, J. J. (1986). Lessons from hospice evaluations: Counterpoint. *The Hospice Journal, 2*, 9–15

Mallett, K., Price, J. H., Jurs, S. G., & Slenker, R. S. (1991). Relationships among burnout, death anxiety, and social support in hospice and critical care nurses. *Psychological Reports, 68*, 1347–1359.

Maloney, C. M., Kesner, R. K., Klein, G., & Bockenstette, J. (1989). The rectal administration of MS Contin: Clinical implications of use in end stage cancer. *American Journal of Hospice Care, 6,* 34–35.

Martens, N., & Davies, B. (1990). The work of patients and spouses in managing advanced cancer at home. *The Hospice Journal, 6,* 55–73.

Martin, T. O. (1982–1983). Death anxiety and social desirability among nurses. *Omega, 13,* 51–58.

Massie, J. J., Holland, J., & Glass, E. (1983). Delirium in terminally ill cancer patients. *American Journal of Psychiatry, 140,* 1048–1050.

Masters, M., & Shontz, F. C. (1989). Identification of problems and strengths of the hospice client by clients, caregivers and nurses. *Cancer Nursing, 12,* 226–235.

McCubbin, H. I., Larsen, A. S., & Olson, D. H. (1982). F-copes family coping strategies. In D. H. Olson, H. I. McCubbin, H. Barnes, A. Larsen, M. Muxen, & M. Wilson (Eds.), *Family inventories* (pp. 101–120). Minneapolis, MN: University of Minnesota.

McGinnis, S. S. (1986). How can nurses improve the quality of life of the hospice client and family?: An exploratory study. *The Hospice Journal, 2,* 23–36.

Melzack, R., Ofiesh, J. G., & Mount, B. M. (1976). The Brompton Mixture: Effects on pain in cancer patients. *Canadian Medical Association Journal, 115,* 125–129.

Mor, V. (1986). Assessing patient outcomes in hospice: What to measure? *The Hospice Journal, 2,* 17–35.

Mor, V. (1987). *Hospice care systems: Structure, process, costs, and outcome.* New York: Springer Publishing Co.

Mor, V., & Laliberte, L. (1984). Burnout among hospice staff. *Health Social Work, 9,* 274–283.

Mor, V., Wachtel, T. J., & Kidder, D. (1985). Patient predictors of hospice choice— hospital versus home care programs. *Medical Care, 23,* 1115–1119.

Morris, J. N., Mor, V., Goldberg, R. J., Sherwood, S., Greer, D. S., & Hiris, J. (1986). The effect of treatment setting and patient characteristics on pain in terminal cancer patients: A report from the National Hospice Society. *Journal of Chronic Diseases, 39,* 26–35.

Moseley, J. R. (1985). Alterations in comfort. *Nursing Clinics of North America, 20,* 427–438.

Mount, B. M. (1978). Palliative care of the terminally ill. Royal College Lecture presented at the *Annual Meeting of the Royal College of Physicians and Surgeons of Canada,* Vancouver, British Columbia, January 27.

Mount, B. M., Ajemian, I., & Scott, J. F. (1976). The use of the Brompton Mixture in treating the chronic pain of malignant disease. *Canadian Medical Association Journal, 115,* 122–124.

National Pressure Ulcer Advisory Panel. (1989). Pressure ulcers prevalence, cost, and risk assessment. Consensus development conference statement. *Decubitus, 2,* 24–28.

Normile, L. B. (1990). Psychological distress in bereavement: A comparative study of parents of adult children who died of cancer versus AIDS. *Dissertation Abstracts International, 50,* 2840. Order No. AAD 89-23121.

O'Brien Abt, M. E. (1983). An identification of the needs of family members of terminally ill patients in a hospital setting. *Military Medicine, 148,* 712–716.

Padilla, G. V., Present, C., Grant, N. M., Metter, G., Lipsett, J., & Heide, F. (1983). Quality of life index for patients with cancer. *Research in Nursing and Health, 83,* 117–126.

Penzel, Y. (1985). Letter to the editor. *Oncology Times, VII.*

Petrosino, B. M. (1986a). Research challenges in hospice nursing. In B. M. Petrosino (Ed.), Nursing in hospice and terminal care: Research and practice, *The Hospice Journal*, 2, 1–10.

Petrosino, B. M. (1986b). "Introduction" Nursing in hospice and terminal care: Research and practice. *The Hospice Journal*, 2, 15–16.

Petrosino, B. M. (1988). Nursing research in hospice care. *The Hospice Journal*, 4, 29–45.

Reuben, D. B., & Mor, V. (1985). Dyspnea in terminal cancer patients. *Chest*, 89, 234–236.

Sanders, C. (1978). Typologies and symptoms of adult bereavement. Doctoral Dissertation, University of South Florida, Tampa, FL.

Saunders, C. (1967). *The management of terminal illness*. London: Hospital Medical Publishing.

Schleifer, S. J., Keller, S. E., Camerino, M., Thornton, J. C., & Stein, M. (1983). Suppression of lymphocyte stimulation following bereavement. *Journal of the American Medical Association*, 250, 374–377.

Seale, C. F. (1989). What happens in hospices: A review of research evidence. *Social Science & Medicine*, 28, 551–559.

Seale, C. F. (1991). A comparison of hospice and conventional care. *Social Science & Medicine*, 32, 147–152.

Shea, J. D. (1975). Pressure sores: Classification and management. *Clinical Orthopedics*, 112, 89–100.

Skorupka, P., & Bohnet, N. (1982). Primary caregivers' perceptions of nursing behaviors that best meet their needs in a home care hospice setting. *Cancer Nursing*, 5, 371–374.

Spiegel, D., Bloom, J. R., Kraemer, H. C., & Gottheil, E. (1989). Effect of psychosocial treatment on survival of patients with metastatic breast cancer. *The Lancet*, 5, 888–891.

Steele, L. L. (1990). The death surround: Factors influencing the grief experience of survivors. *Oncology Nursing Forum*, 17, 235–241.

Torrens, P. R. (1986). U.S. hospice between two worlds: Economic realities and patient care needs. *Journal of Palliative Care*, 2, 6–8.

Twycross, R. G. (1979). Clinical experience with diamorphine in advanced malignant disease. *International Journal of Clinical Pharmacology, Therapy and Toxicology*, 9, 184–198.

Twycross, R. G. 1977. Choice of strong analgesic in terminal cancer: Diamorphine or morphine? *Pain*, 3, 93–104.

Twycross, R. G. (1983). Principles and practice of pain relief in terminal cancer. In C. Corr & D. Corr (Eds.), *Hospice care: Principles and practice* (pp. 55–72). New York: Springer Publishing Co.

Wachtel, T., Allen-Masterson, S., Reuben, D., Goldberg, R., & Mor, V. (1988). The end stage cancer patient: Terminal common pathway. *The Hospice Journal*, 4, 43–80.

Wald, F. S., Foster, Z., & Wald, H. J. (1980). The hospice movement as a health care reform. *Nursing Outlook*, 28, 171–178.

Walsh, T. D. (1990). Continuing care in a medical center: The Cleveland Clinic Foundation Palliative Care Service. *Journal of Pain and Symptom Management*, 5, 273–278.

Wegmann, J. A. (1987). Hospice home death, hospital death and coping abilities of widows. *Cancer Nursing*, 10, 148–155.

Wickham, R. (1989). Managing chemotherapy-related nausea and vomiting: The state of the art. *Oncology Nursing Forum*, 16, 563–574.

PART III
Research on Nursing Education

Chapter 7

Research on the Baccalaureate Completion Process for RNs

Mary Beth Mathews
Riverside Methodist Hospitals

Lucille L. Travis
Frances Payne Bolton School of Nursing
Case Western Reserve University

CONTENTS

This chapter provides a review of research-based literature for the decade 1983–1993 on the registered nurse (RN) as a prospective or current student in a baccalaureate nursing program in the U.S. Such programs facilitate access to the bachelor's degree in nursing for RNs within the same, a parallel, or a separate educational track as generic nursing students, or in a program specifically designed for the RN. The latter such programs are called by such descriptors as "completion programs," "2 plus 2 programs," and "second step" programs.

Two previous research reviews provided guidance for the decisions made about materials to include in this review (Holzemer, 1983; Schwirian, 1985). Two of the eight chapters in the first reference deal with research conducted to that date related to RNs as BSN students, primarily their characteristics as compared to generic students (Baj, 1983; Watson, 1983). One of the four areas recommended by Schwirian (1985) for future research on nursing students was "second step" programs, specifically to provide "empirical evidence as to what educators *do* and what they *should do* (p. 227). The purpose of this integrative research review is to provide a summary of that empirical evidence to inform decisions about and recommend future research direction for RN/BSN education.

To identify studies for the review, computerized searches using the Cumulative Index to Nursing and Allied Health Literature (CINAHL) and MEDLINE were conducted for inclusive years 1983 through 1993. Terms used alone and in combination for the search included Education, Nursing, Baccalaureate; Registered Nurses; Students, Nursing; Students or Education, -Post-RN; Re-entry Students; and Students, Nontraditional. Guided by the CINAHL printout, the authors obtained and reviewed journal articles appearing by article title to be relevant to the research review, which had been published in refereed nursing journals. The search was then extended to the citations provided by authors of the research reports found to be relevant and to DISSERTATION ABSTRACTS (on CD-ROM discs), Academic Abstracts and the ERIC database. Research reports using non-U.S. samples (e.g., Canadian, Australian) were excluded as were all unpublished doctoral dissertations. Research reports containing all of the following components were reviewed: research theme or focus; type of research design (e.g., exploratory/descriptive, experimental, phenomenological); elements of design (sampling, methods, analysis of data); and key findings. Studies meeting the criteria reflected three general themes of inquiry: (a) characteristics descriptive of RNs as BSN students, and as compared to generic students; (b) program outcome achievement by RNs as BSN students, and as compared to generic students; and (c) programmatic variations in relation to recruitment, retention, and successful graduation of RN–BSN students. The scope of the review is limited to existing published reports of research and program evaluations meeting the criteria. Excluded, therefore, are numerous unpublished doctoral dissertations and nonempirical reports of RN/BSN program practices that did not meet requisite criteria of this review.

The findings of the authors are similar to those of Schwirian (1985) in the following respects: (a) changes of attitudes in self-concept and professionalism can be attributed to nursing school program participation; (b) with few exceptions, studies reviewed used nonrandom, small, single-site convenience samples with the result that the generalizability of study findings is limited; (c) as research on nursing students remains largely problem-driven, it is generally fragmented and noncumulative; and (d) there remains the need to develop valid, reliable measures of desired professional practice behaviors and to develop and test models through which such practice behaviors can be developed in both generic and RN/BSN students.

RESEARCH RELATED TO CHARACTERISTICS OF STUDENTS

The majority of the studies of RNs as BSN students prior to 1983 considered descriptive characteristics, usually in comparison with a cohort of generic students. Since that time, researchers have investigated a wider range of variables. Seventeen studies will be reviewed here related to such avenues of inquiry as demographics, attitudes toward nursing, interpersonal and personality characteristics including self-concept, characteristics as learners, and well-being characteristics (stress, anxiety, and coping strategies).

Descriptive Characteristics

Using a descriptive survey design, Baj (1985) compared a sample of 251 RN and generic baccalaureate students from 12 programs in California on 24 variables such as age, marital status, and number of dependents, financial status, prior vocational experience, and recent major life events. She found the majority of BSN students to be part-time students and full-time employees in contrast with their generic student counterparts. The RN was generally married or divorced, had one or more children, was employed full-time as a staff nurse in the acute care settings, and was not receiving financial aid. Generic students, in contrast, tended to be younger, single, or recently married, not working, or working part time while attending school full time, and receiving some type of financial assistance. These findings reinforce those published between 1971 and 1982, that RN and generic students have different demographic characteristics that should be taken into account by generic baccalaureate programs in design and implementation of curricula and program implementation policies. Baj recommended research on the impact of such supportive interventions as flexible scheduling, provisions for meeting child care needs, and special needs of RN students who may experience separation, divorce, or a child-care crisis.

   Thurber (1988) compared the differences in attitudes toward professional nursing between generic and RN/BSN completion students from a convenience sample of 233 students from one geographic area. The cross-sectional design allowed for evaluation of students at the time of entrance and exit from programs. Both groups were highly motivated academic achievers and were interested in career advancement and access to higher educational opportunities. On program completion both groups demonstrated gains in professional attitudes as well as similar exit program expectations. From the comparison, Thurber suggested examining creative methods to provide programs to greater benefit these students.

Using a small convenient sample and a longitudinal study design, Krouse (1988) compared personality characteristics of beginning RN/BSN students and beginning diploma students at three timepoints: entry, midway, and end of the program. Evaluating the results from the California Psychological Inventory (Gough, 1957; Megargee, 1972) she found the RNs were different from the traditional diploma school students in the areas of leadership potential and intellectual ability. RN/BSN students were mature, forceful, aggressive, independent, and showed leadership potential; on the other hand, diploma graduates who were not enrolled in a BSN program were more likely to be impatient, inhibited, unsure, submissive, and even manipulative in personality trait. As a result of this study, Krouse recommended that RN curricula be designed to enhance the assertiveness of the RN student.

A number of researchers examined interpersonal characteristics of enrolled RN students. Rendon (1988) used a localized convenience sample of 167 RNs enrolled in five BSN programs, who completed The Cohen CAD scale (Cohen, 1967) and the Rendon Perceptions of Student Role (PSR) scale (1988), to measure the degree of congruence between interpersonal orientation and perceptions of the student role of the RN/BSN student. She found that those students with high compliant interpersonal orientations had congruence in their student role. Those students with detached orientations had incongruence in their student role. One of the more interesting conclusions of this study was that the majority of students expressed a strong commitment and determination in their student role, however. As a result of this study, Rendon recommended a number of activities for both the faculty and students to enhance the RN/BSN learning experience.

Another direction for research on student characteristics is reflected in the work of King (1986, 1988), who examined differences and similarities among RN and generic nursing students from the perspective of adult development theory. Specifically, the study measured life stage, ego development, and learning styles as a measure of individual adult development, which, in turn, was correlated with participation in higher education and perceived importance of education for adult development. Convenience samples of RN students and generic students enrolled in a baccalaureate nursing program of a large state-supported university were obtained. Instrumentation included the University of Washington Sentence Completion test (UWSCT) to measure ego development (Loevinger & Wessler, 1970), the Kolb Learning Style Inventory (KSLI) (Kolb, 1974), and the Tarule's Educational Experience Inventory (EEI) (Weathersby, 1977) to measure life phases and the impact of education on adult development. For the first study (1986), King stated null hypotheses. She found similar demographic differences between student groups to those of Baj (1985). Further, RN and generic students were similar with respect to learning styles and differed significantly on ego development (perceptions, interpretations) and life stage. With respect to the latter, King concluded that generic students were in Early Adult Transition, whereas the RN–BSN students were in either the Age 30 Transition or the Mid-Life Transition stages. In a second study, King (1988) used the same instrumentation to test directional hypotheses and found similar differences between RN and generic baccalaureate students. The RNs were focused on career development opportunities and the degree of program satisfaction for all students appeared to be directly related to one's adult development stage. Although limited in their generalizability because of the single site convenience sample design, these two studies point the direction for further exploration of the differences and similarities among RN and generic students on variables more substantive than demographics.

Using a convenience sample of 175 generic and 170 RN–BSN students, Linares (1989) compared the learning characteristics of junior level students in two state-supported baccalaureate schools of nursing in one state. The following instrumentation was used for data collection: the Adult Nowicki-Strickland Internal-External Scale (ANS-IE) (Nowicki & Duke, 1974) in which the higher the score, the more external the subject's locus of control; the Learning Preference Inventory (LPI) (Rezler & Rezmovic, 1981) in which scores on subscales reflect relative preference for that learning style; and the Self-Directed Learning Readiness Scale (SDLRS) (Guglielmino, 1980), which scores readiness for self-directed learning from low to high readiness. There were no significant differences between the two samples with respect to the three constructs. Age had a statistically significant positive influence on readiness for self-directed learning, however.

Shepherd and Brooks (1991) used the Tennessee Self-Concept Scale (Fitts, 1965) to compare levels of self-concept among a convenience sample of associate degree, diploma, generic baccalaureate, and upper-division baccalaureate nursing students in southeastern Pennsylvania; they found no statistically significant differences in the measure of self-concept among the four types of senior students.

Well-being of Students

Nearly a decade ago the need for research related to the health of nursing students was identified, that is, student concerns, stress, and anxiety (Schwirian, 1985). Several studies have focused on the impact of school on the RNs as students. Derstine (1988) examined sources of stress or anxiety for RNs as BSN students. Using a convenience sample of 203 RN students from the Philadelphia area, Derstine (1988) measured anxiety of students at the beginning of their program of study. She compared the results of selected demographic data and trait anxiety scores from the Spielberger's State Trait Anxiety Inventory (1983). From a stepwise multiple regression of trait anxiety in the demographic variables, three predictors of trait anxiety were identified: nursing program type, being married, and being separated. In particular, diploma graduates had lower trait anxiety scores than did associate-degree graduates; and those students who were married or separated had greater trait anxiety scores than did unmarried students. Derstine suggested that RN educators note such demographic variables of students to identify those students at risk for anxiety.

Beck and Srivastava (1991) examined perceived level of stress and sources of stress during participation in a baccalaureate nursing program. A convenience sample of 67 generic and 25 RN/BSN students enrolled in one nursing program was used. Three instruments were used to collect the data: (a) the General Health Questionnaire (GHQ) to measure general distress and minor psychiatric disorders (Banks, 1983; Goldberg, 1972); (b) the Stress Inventory, a combination of the Stress Incident Record (Firth & Morrison, 1985) and the stress scales of Firth (1986) and of Frances and Naftel (1983); and (c) a demographic profile sheet. The stress scores for all students were significantly higher than for the population in general, whereas those for the RN/BSN students were significantly lower than for the generic students.

Both Lee (1988) and Mattson (1990) examined coping strategies of RNs while BSN students. Using a sample of 111 students from four schools located in the southern part of California, Lee found that 82% of the re-entry students used direct action as a coping method in dealing with stress. In another study of coping, Mattson (1990) used two instruments to measure maturity and coping: (a) Way of Coping (Folkman & Lazarus, 1985), and the Student Developmental Task Inventory-2nd edition (SDTI-2) (Winston, Miller, & Prince, 1979). From a convenience sample of 138 RN students in one completion program, the three coping strategies used most frequently by successful students were "social support," "being problem-focused," and "being positive-focused." In addition, the effective copers had higher scores on developmental maturity than did ineffective ones. Ineffective copers more often chose "self-blame," "wishful thinking," and "self-isolation" as coping strategies. As a result of this study, Mattson (1990) suggested that RN students be encouraged to improve their problem-solving skills and use support systems for assistance.

A further examination of stress and coping by RN students, as elicited by the variables of burnout, lifestress, and support for returning to school, was completed by Dick and Anderson (1993). Using a convenience sample of 53 RN students, burnout was measured using the Maslach Burnout Inventory (Maslach & Jackson, 1986). Life stress was measured with the Schedule of Recent Experiences Scale (Holmes & Rahe, 1967), and support for returning to school was measured by an instrument developed by the authors. The findings indicated that the burnout experienced by the RN student was no higher than reported among nurses in clinical practice (Topf & Dillon, 1988). In addition, there were no significant relationships between burnout and increased life events stress, or time commitments for work and school. As support from colleagues and family increased, burnout decreased, however. Therefore, the authors suggested that educators encourage students to consciously build or optimize their personal support systems and that institutions design mechanisms to increase support for students returning to school.

RESEARCH RELATED TO
PROGRAM OUTCOME ACHIEVEMENT

Only six published studies were found relating to the achievement of program outcomes by RN/BSN students. All studies addressed the concept of professionalism or professionalization of the RN/BSN student. Two studies examined the relationship of professionalization to the development of critical thinking competence of RN/BSN students. Throwe and Fought (1987) described the theoretical framework for and the elements of a tool used in one nursing program for the formative and summative evaluation of the socialization process of the RN/BSN student through the program and upon degree completion. Their work should be useful for research by others.

Professionalization/Socialization

Whelan (1984) studied the effect of a senior-level course on the degree of professionalism demonstrated by RN/BSN students, using a sample of entering students and graduating senior students. Instrumentation was provided by Corwin's role-orientation instrument (Corwin, 1961) as modified by Dr. M. E. Devis. Whelan found that graduates held a role orientation that was less bureaucratic, more professional, and more service-oriented than was the role orientation of entering nursing students.

Lawler and Rose (1987) used a descriptive ex post facto design to determine if there were differences in professionalization (a measure of professional socialization) among ADN, BSN, and RN/BSN students. A nonprobability purposive sampling technique was used to obtain three homogeneous groups at the same point in time (within 2–3 weeks of graduation), and the researchers used two instruments for data collection: Stone's Health Care Professional Attitude Inventory (Stone & Knopke, 1978) as modified by Lawler and Rose (1987), and Corwin's Nursing Role Conception Scale (Corwin, 1961). Lawler and Rose (1987) found that RN/BSN students scored higher on the measure of professionalism than did either generic BSN or ADN students. RN/BSN students also exhibited more congruence between ideal and actual professional role behaviors than did either generic RN or ADN students. The researchers concluded that RNs could achieve program outcomes of baccalaureate education at or above the same levels as generic students. Periard, Bell, Knecht, and Woodman (1991) studied changes in professional attitudes of RN/BSN students over the course of the BSN program as a measure of professional socialization. Using a cross-sectional design and a multistage cluster sample of 296 students from NLN-accredited nursing programs in four midwestern states, the researchers measured trust, intolerance of ambiguity, self-concept, and professional goals. They found a significant increase in professional attitudes, confirming that RNs advanced toward professionalism during their educational program, and that trust, intolerance of ambiguity, self-concept, and professional goals were significantly related to professional attitudes. The authors recommended that faculty model professionalism as defined in each program, and suggested the elements of professionalism be systematically addressed in curriculum design, teaching strategies and for advising and counseling.

Hughes, Wade, and Peters (1991) investigated the perception of role competencies and development of self-concept among a convenience sample of 4 RNs and 70 generic BSN students from one program. As part of a one-group pretest–posttest design, students completed the Tennessee Self-Concept Scale (Fitts, 1965) and the Slater Nursing Competencies Rating Scale (Wandelt, 1975). The major finding was that a senior-level synthesis course had a positive impact on self-esteem of senior professional nurses, and that all students experienced an increase in their self-concept and role competency scores. Although the sample size was so small as to preclude meaningful comparison of generic and RN/BSN scores, the authors concluded that learning experiences can be intentionally designed, which will result in greater self-confidence and a greater self-concept for baccalaureate nursing students, including registered nurses.

Professionalization and Critical Thinking

As of 1993 baccalaureate nursing competencies required by the National League for Nursing will include critical thinking, communication, and therapeutic intervention. The assessment of critical thinking as a desired outcome of baccalaureate education and as related to creative thinking and to nursing performance was the focus of Sullivan's work (1987) with RNs who return to school. An intact purposive sample of 51 RNs enrolled in one midwestern university RN/BSN program was obtained. Measurement instruments included the Watson-Glaser Critical Thinking Appraisal to assess critical thinking (CTA, forms A and B, Watson & Glaser, 1964); the Torrance Test of Creative Thinking (TTCT, verbal forms A & B) to assess creative ability (Torrance & Torrance, 1974); and the Stewart Evaluation of Nursing Scale (SS) to evaluate nursing performance (Slater-Stewart, 1979). Data collection occurred at two times: in the first 4 weeks of the first semester of the BSN program, and in the last 4 weeks of the students' final semester in the program. Data were analyzed using a t-test to compare mean scores on all measures upon program entry and completion; intercorrelations among subject scores on all three instruments were obtained using Pearson's Product Moment Correlation. In comparing scores on program completion with those on entry, the researcher found that overall creativity scores were lower, critical thinking scores showed no difference, and clinical performance, verbal flexibility, and grade point average were significantly higher. These conclusions must be interpreted cautiously as they reflect results for one group of students within one program of study, and may be associated with other variables not considered. The study design should be helpful for nurse educators who must develop methods to measure and to document program outcomes for RNs in baccalaureate nursing programs, however.

Brooks and Shepherd (1992) linked the assessment of professionalism and critical thinking in their study of senior nursing students in four types of nursing programs. Following an excellent summary of the significance of RN/BSN education for the profession's goal of preparing professionals for practice, the authors clearly set forth their research questions, study methods, and summary of data analysis. The purpose of the study was to determine if there were correlations between critical thinking and professionalism among the four types of students and educational programs. The convenience sample of 200 persons, comprised of 50 students each from ADN, diploma, generic baccalaureate, and RN/BSN student groups, was obtained from NLN-accredited programs in one eastern state. Instrumentation included the Watson-Glaser Critical Thinking Appraisal or WHCTA (Watson & Glaser, 1964) to assess critical thinking ability, and the Health Care Professional Attitude Inventory (HCPAI, Stone & Knopke, 1978) to assess level of professionalism achieved. The researchers found that there was a strong positive correlation between critical thinking ability and levels of professionalism for the combined sample, and the researchers recommend that an increased emphasis on critical thinking skills be initiated across all nursing programs. They also found that critical thinking abilities of senior RN/BSN and generic students were almost identical, and were significantly higher than either diploma or ADN students. Senior RN/BSN students also achieved higher professionalism scores than any other group, and there was no significant difference between levels of professionalism exhibited by seniors in generic and in ADN programs. Further, senior diploma nursing students exhibited the lowest professionalism of the four samples, and the researchers posited as a variable for further study an association with the bureaucratic and hierarchical environment in which socialization is occurring for those students. This study does suggest that the outcomes RNs can attain through

RN/BSN curricula are comparable to generic 4-year programs with respect to the two variables of professionalism level and critical thinking ability. These findings were obtained from a single study using a convenience sample of volunteer students and a posttest format, however. No assessments were made of proficiency on program entry nor of the potential influence of faculty on the development of professionalism.

RESEARCH RELATED TO PROGRAMMATIC VARIATIONS IN RN-BSN EDUCATION

Twelve articles were reviewed for this category, and at least 10 additional articles were excluded because they were descriptive reports of current program practices rather than research-based reports. The majority of the literature in this category related to recruitment and progression of students, including practices related to the validation of prior knowledge and skill and to program articulation. It also was related to programmatic characteristics associated with satisfaction, socialization, and achievement of the RN in BSN programs.

Program Selection Factors

Specific motivational aspects of the RNs' decision to pursue their BSN degree was examined by Fotos (1987). In a survey of 57 students who completed a modified version of the Educational Participation Scale (Boshier, 1973; O'Connor, 1979), Fotos found that RNs were motivated most to pursue the degree by a desire for professional advancement. In addition, a majority of students were not in the mainstream of campus life and were beyond the traditional age of college students. As a result of the study, Fotos suggested strategies for faculty in curriculum planning and advisement.

To position the nursing program in the most advantageous position in an increasingly competitive market with a declining student application pool, Rawlins, Riordan, Delamaide, and Kilian (1991) conducted a study to identify factors that influenced program selection by students and program graduates, determine relevant market segments, and identify factors thought to be most effective in reaching prospects. For this market research, the sample was comprised of 87 students and 141 alumni of a small, private nursing college. The mail survey instrument was developed by a marketing consultant in cooperation with the nursing faculty. Personal contact by direct mail or talking with the nurse recruiter were cited as the most important influence on developing awareness about the nursing program. Canonical correlation analysis (CCA) of demographics and program type (independent set) and items influencing the decision to attend (dependent set) was used to segment students and alumni into two distinct market segments: nontraditional/traditional, and transfer/local. The traditional students (under 25 years of age, unmarried, local) chose a BSN program due to the quality of clinical instruction and availability of financial aid. Nontraditional students, on the other hand (age 25 or older, married, returning RN in BSN program) chose a program primarily on the basis of convenience. For both groups personal contact with a nurse recruiter for the program was a very important factor influencing selection decisions. Discriminant analysis was used following the CCA to determine differences within those two groups. Traditional students were most influenced to attend by perceptions of the institution and its faculty; nontraditional students were most influenced to attend by special programs for returning students, class schedule, geographic location to home/work and small size of college.

An avenue of inquiry has been the determinants of program selection for RNs who do enroll in RN/BSN programs. In a sample of 1268 RN respondents (50.3% response rate), Lange (1986) identified variables predictive of enrollment in RN/BSN program. The four variables were: (a) currently enrolled in an academic course; (b) expressed a high level of interest in obtaining a BSN; (c) inquired about BSN programs; and (d) had previously earned academic credit. Lange found that RNs with intent to enroll in the BSN program are more apt to be younger, associate degree nursing program graduates, currently enrolled in an academic course for credit, have a high interest in obtaining a BSN, and to have earned previous academic credit. The RNs intending to enroll are highly motivated, more achievement oriented, take initiative to obtain information for career decision making, and in general expect the BSN to increase job options in the future. Specific recommendations for recruitment, pre-enrollment advisement, student support group formation, and program content are offered.

Validation and Progression Strategies

Validation is the process by which previous learning is assessed for the purpose of giving credit or placing the student in an advanced level of a course or program. Competency examination (texting) is one strategy used to assess and give credit for prior education and experience. The most common tests used for this purpose in RN-BSN education are ACT-PEP examinations. Yang and Noble (1990) initiated a study in fall 1984 to determine the validity of the ACT-PEP tests for predicting the academic performance of RNs in BSN programs. Thirty of the 33 nursing institutions selected from those national institutions who had received at least 50 ACT-PEP reports during the previous academic year agreed to participate. Following computation of descriptive statistics, multiple regression prediction equations were developed and run for each institution for each ACT-PEP test. Across institutions, student demographic characteristics did not contribute to the explanation of academic performance beyond that accounted for by the ACT-PEP test scores. The single most important variable in predicting academic performance was found to be the ACT-PEP test score. The authors offer some cautionary remarks about generalizability. In particular, it is possible that age and test scores were correlated such that age offered no additional information after score had been entered into the regression.

In a more recent study, Kearney (1991) considered the relationship between performance on a standardized validation examination and performance in required course work in the nursing program. Using record review and a convenience sample of all RN graduates of a single BSN program (n = 182), Kearney found that RN students scored higher on validation exams the longer the interval since graduation from a diploma program. High performance on validation exams also was significantly associated with good performance on prerequisite and concurrent science coursework in the BSN program.

The RN brings practice experience as well as knowledge to the BSN program. Long and Redding (1991) initiated the development and evaluation of a clinical performance examination for validating clinical skills of RNs entering a baccalaureate nursing program. The researchers completed a pilot study of the instrument but were incomplete in their reporting of both their method and results.

Oechsle, Volden, and Lambeth (1990) conducted a summative evaluation of the use of portfolios with RN BSN students as a mechanism for validating previous knowledge and skill. The sample for the study was 34 RNs who chose to develop a portfolio for partial or complete credit for professional nursing leadership and management in the BSN program at one western college of nursing. A mailed survey was used for data collection. Part one requested demographic data, the second section elicited reasons why the RNs returned to school for the BSN, and the third section was 12 yes/no questions about the RNs' experience with the portfolio validation process. The authors found that: (1) the approach reinforced adult learning theory, self-directed learning, and commitment to summative evaluation procedures; (2) 87% of the respondents found the process to be fair; and (3) most were satisfied with the amount of credit awarded. Following a discussion of strengths and weaknesses of the portfolio approach to validation of prior learning with one sample of learners in one setting, the authors recommended that guidelines be developed to assist nurse educators to use this mechanism.

In a retrospective study replicating work by Allen, Higgs, and Holloway (1988), Kroll (1990) sought to determine predictors of success of RNs in BSN education. He analyzed the academic records of 81 students admitted over a 4-year period to an integrated baccalaureate nursing program in one northwestern university. Sixteen of those students did not complete the program, but the remaining 65 finished within a 4-year period. For this sample of students the correlation between success on challenge exams and high GPA was statistically significant. Further, GPA on previous college course work was also predictive of program success, whereas demographic variables such as age, experience, and number of years out of school were not.

Program Variations and RN Satisfaction

Lee (1987) compared stressful didactic and clinical experiences for a sample of 40 RN students enrolled in generic baccalaureate nursing programs and 71 students in RN-only programs. The samples were from nursing programs located in the southern part of California. In general, didactic experiences rather than clinical experiences generated stress for the RN students, specifically the variable of inadequate instruction. In contrast, generic students identified the didactic stress as examinations, grades, and pressures of schedules. Lee suggested that nurse educators be aware of incidents that produce stress in RN students so that they can adjust their instruction appropriately.

From her study of program characteristics most satisfying for students enrolled in different types of baccalaureate programs, Beeman (1988) found that RNs in RN-only programs found the programs to be most supportive of their practice autonomy, whereas RNs in less traditional programs found less flexibility and more limitations on professional initiative. Beeman's sample of 284 undergraduate nursing students from 12 BSN programs in a western state included 188 RNs. Instrumentation used to collect program information was the Beeman Educational Environment Measure for Adult Nurses (BEEMAN) developed by the author, which included a demographic data section, five open-ended questions about choice of program and satisfaction with program, and 73 attitudinal statements about various facets of the baccalaureate educational environment. Although RNs in both generic and RN-only programs found the program met their adult learning needs, RNs in generic programs expressed the most need for change in their educational environment, specifically related to cost and repeated program content. Beeman found program satisfaction to be an important factor in RN success in BSN education, and that satisfaction is enhanced by faculty understanding of student differences, use of learning strategies that foster self-direction and acquisition of practical knowledge, and accommodation for student variations in levels of professional socialization and development. This was a large, well-designed study and the findings suggest the importance of addressing the unique learning needs of RNs as adults when the RN/BSN students are integrated with generic students in one program of study.

Baker and Barlow (1988), evaluated a self-paced baccalaureate program for RNs. They found that program flexibility, excellent learning resources, and peer interaction were factors promoting success for 89 (50%) of the 178 graduates surveyed. Student characteristics associated with success were positive motivation to succeed, determination and self-direction, and the presence of family support. Eighty-eight percent of the respondents indicated that they had financial concerns that needed to be resolved before they could begin a BSN program, and that flexible work scheduling, support of fellow employees and the opportunity to work part-time contributed significantly to their progression success. Further, characteristics of the faculty that graduates viewed as important for student success included encouragement about progress and being supportive, recognition of student background, and the qualities of consideration, caring, and friendliness. Of least importance to the students was the content expertise of the faculty, a finding that was contrary to previous findings reported in the literature.

Another researcher found that the program characteristics needed by RNs to facilitate their success in the BSN program are directly related to their personal characteristics (Wang, 1991). Using a convenience sample of 94 RNs in one NLN-accredited upper division BSN program, the researcher conducted content analysis of 245 critical incidents provided by the RNs to identify and analyze stressful and satisfying educational experiences that these learners documented. The theoretical framework for the study was the transactional conceptual model of adult education developed by Boyd and Apps (1980), in which factors helping or hindering individual adult learning are determined. Among the findings were that RN students provided almost twice as many stressful as satisfying incidents for analysis with many of those relating to scheduling of courses and clinical activities. Interpersonal relationships were among the sources most frequently cited as satisfying educational experiences for all students. Although limited in generalizability because of the single site small sample size design, this study's findings support adult learning theory as an appropriate framework for regarding RN–BSN students.

McClelland and Daly (1991), using a sample of 72 RN students from one campus and a satellite site of one midwestern university, compared demographic characteristics and learning achievement of on-campus and satellite-site learners. They found a significant difference in certain demographic characteristics and academic performance between RNs on a satellite campus and those on the central campus. Specifically, satellite campus students took significantly longer to complete the program, worked significantly more hours, and drove further to attend class, and had significantly more children than did on-campus students. The satellite campus RN-BSN students also performed better on the ACT-PEP examinations as compared to on-campus students, however. The author recommends the use of the latest telecommunications technology for delivering educational courses to on-campus and satellite sites, and flexible course scheduling in light of the fact that the majority of the learners are working full time and have families. This single-site small sample study provides a contribution to support alternate site delivery of education to meet the needs of adult learners.

In a related study, Viverais-Dresler and Kutschke (1992) examined the satisfaction of students with clinical teaching of introductory nursing courses offered by distance education technology. From a sample of 98 female RN students who had completed the three-course sequence, 41 (44%) completed a mailed questionnaire. Overall satisfaction levels were no lower than 72% (related to assistance with writing assignments) and was as high as 100% (e.g., fairness of grading and of clinical evaluation). Recommendations for improvement, however, were in the areas of increasing structured instruction early in the course, and coaching in self-direction skills. Further research is recommended to facilitate generalizability of the findings from this one-sample, single-site study, and to examine further the incongruence between expressed needs of RN students as learners and the accepted principles of adult education.

Program Articulation

Systematic evaluation of articulation project experiences is necessary to inform policy decisions for nursing programs, state educational boards, and national professional societies. With respect to articulation between types of RN programs, Deleruyelle and Chally (1984) surveyed by mail 139 BSN programs in the US, including 46 in the north-central Midwest, regarding their articulation policies for RNs in BSN programs. When comparing their findings to those of Petrone (1977), they found that, although there was no uniformity, there was a trend emerging in the field toward establishing policies for validating previous knowledge and skill, and for evaluating clinical competence.

McHugh (1991) investigated the educational validity of direct articulation for Associate-Degree Nursing (ADN) graduates into one upper division RN/BSN program in an eastern university, as an alternate strategy to the use of proficiency examinations to validate previous knowledge. In Phase #1 of the study the objectives and content of the university's ACT-PEP nursing validation battery was compared to the philosophy, goals, objectives, and content of four ADN feeder schools to identify a common core of content in both ADN and BSN programs. Areas of omission were identified. In Phase #2 of the study, the ACT-PEP battery of tests were administered to 425 ADN students 1 week prior to graduation. McHugh obtained a direct relationship between end-of-program GPA and the graduate's composite mean on the ACT-PEP validation battery, and no significant difference in composite mean scores among students anticipating transfer to the upper division BSN program. Based on the findings, one university established a policy permitting transfer of lower division nursing credit in lieu of completion of the ACT-PEP validation battery for ADN candidates with a GPA of 2.75 or higher.

The Maryland Statewide Articulation Model was one of the first statewide approaches to facilitating educational mobility for RNs prepared in associate degree and diploma programs. Rapson, Perry, and Parker (1990) implemented a study to determine whether there is a difference in educational outcomes for RNs who choose different advanced placement pathways available in the Maryland model: direct transfer, advanced placement examination, or nursing transition course. Educational outcome was defined as the score on the NLN Comprehensive Nursing Achievement Test (CNAT) for Baccalaureate Nursing Students, and grades from two clinical courses taken the previous two academic semesters. The sample used were 113 RNs enrolled in the clinical concepts courses at the University of Maryland, the prerequisites for which are successful completion of one of the three articulation processes. Specifically, 15 students had taken the transition course, 41 were direct transfers, and 57 had completed advanced placement examinations. Data analysis was by means of descriptive statistics and analysis of variance between mode of entry and NLN examination scores. Rapson et al. (1990) found that there were no significant differences in performance on the CNAT based on mode of entry to the BSN program; however, students who had completed a transition course performed significantly better in the clinical concepts course than did RN-BSN students who selected other entry routes. Although these findings should increase the confidence of nurse educators to facilitate RN access to the BSN degree, caution should be taken in generalizing the findings because of the disparate sizes of the samples used in this preliminary study.

METHODOLOGICAL AND SUBSTANTIVE ISSUES

Most of the studies reviewed used a convenience sampling method, small sample size, and a limited geographic area from which the sample was drawn. Although the measurement tools used to examine the variety of concepts generally had established reliability and validity, the results of the studies have limited generalizability because of sampling weaknesses. Replication of studies using randomized samples not limited to one geographic location is recommended.

The substantive issues include a dearth of theory-driven research. While adult learning theory is weakly used in some studies, there is little or no theory testing work and it is overstating the state of the art to call any of the studies theory-driven. Most of them are atheoretical or mention a theory in passing. Much of the work seems more like needs assessments than legitimate research. The needs assessments relate primarily to those projects that attempted to find recruitment or retention variables. Such studies appear to be very pragmatic in their goals and study methods.

SUMMARY AND DIRECTIONS FOR FUTURE RESEARCH

Early research on RNs and the baccalaureate degree focused on demographic characteristics of students so as to be instructive to receiving programs (primarily generic baccalaureate programs that were "facilitating" the progression of the RN to the BSN degree within the generic curriculum). Study after study compared RNs and generic students with respect to personal and educational learning need differences. Emphasis was placed on understanding how to apply adult education theory to the design of curricula and the management of clinical experiences. In the mid-1980s the focus of studies then shifted to the identification of variables that were associated with recruitment of RNs to BSN programs, and with their achievement of program outcomes. Educators began sharing in the literature descriptive accounts of program strategies they found to be associated with success for RN students. At about the same time, however, research funding priorities shifted away from education and toward practice; by 1991 clinical outcomes research was being emphasized even for educators, and studies of students and of educational processes became rare indeed.

What can be said about the characteristics of RNs as BSN students, especially when compared to generic students? The studies reviewed attempted to address a number of important characteristics related to RN/BSN students such as: stress, coping strategies, and self-concept. There is evidence that RN and generic BSN students are different with respect to financial responsibilities, educational motivation, and competing demands such as work schedule conflicts. Further research is suggested as to the usefulness of supportive interventions for nonacademic concerns of RNs, with one consideration being that by 1994 RN/BSN students will probably be more similar than different from generic students. Many generic students are second-career individuals; they are older students with families and work responsibilities.

Are there differences between RN/BSN students and generic students with respect to program outcomes? Yes, some differences were found to be related to personality and motivation for education and practice. RNs in baccalaureate education—whether integrated in generic programs or enrolled in RN-only programs—have demonstrated their ability to achieve the same program outcomes of critical thinking and professionalization as their generic RN colleagues.

What programmatic variations are recommended for RN/BSN education that are associated with RN-BSN student success? Validation of prior learning in a manner that acknowledges the adulthood of the RN and facilitates learning and growth rather than duplication and frustration is recommended. Articulation agreements are being developed between types of programs to facilitate the most efficient movement of the RN to the next level of learning if desired.

Most of the studies reviewed used a convenient sampling method, small sample size, and a limited geographic area from which they drew their sample.

Although the measurement tools used to examine the variety of concepts generally has established reliability and validity, the results of the studies have limited generalizability. Replications of studies that use randomized samples not limited to one geographic location are recommended.

Findings of most of the studies support the assertion that generic BSN students and RN/BSN students are more alike than different and can achieve comparable program outcomes. Although there are numerous drawbacks to the comparison of educational programs (Rose, 1988), such findings provide support for the continuation of RN-BSN programs as one means by which the nursing profession can "professionalize" its practitioner resources.

Replication of studies about demographic characteristics of students probably are not warranted. Replication seems indicated for studies related to program outcome achievement (Brooks & Shepherd, 1992; Sullivan, 1987), however. One implication from their work is that practice experience can both facilitate and impede the development of professionalism and critical thinking, in relation to the bureaucratic and hierarchical environment of a hospital. A limited number of databased studies were found that examined curriculum design or student outcomes related to critical thinking, therapeutic intervention, communication, and professionalism.

A second area recommended for inquiry is the impact of baccalaureate education on the practice of the RN following RN/BSN program completion. Of those who go back to school, what happens in their clinical practice? What impact does baccalaureate education have on the patient receiving care from the RN/BSN graduate? Chornick (1992) found that RN/BSN graduates performed critical nursing activities as frequently as graduates of generic BSN programs, and that they performed significantly more behaviors indicating commitment to the profession (i.e., certification, continuing education, additional formal education). Witt (1992) found that RN/BSN graduates had an enhanced self-concept, were less accepting of the oppressed status of nursing in the workplace, and were more apt to join the professional organization than were RNs who did not pursue the BSN. A further area of inquiry could be a comparison of RN/BSN graduates with RNs who get their baccalaureate in another field. Are these groups different from one another as practitioners? If so, on what dimensions? Are their patient care outcomes different? As mentioned several times, there are many descriptive reports in the literature of practices of educators in RN/BSN programs (i.e., Rice, 1992). The authors recommend the intentional use of research methods in program evaluation studies for the purpose of knowledge generation to inform RN/BSN educator practice. As clinical outcomes research is where the funding is, educational research must be funded from foundations and private sponsors. Formation of an interest group among RN/BSN educators could facilitate planning and implementation of a research agenda with multiple sites engaged in the same study to facilitate generalizability of findings.

The North American Society, led by state boards of higher education, is moving away from 2-year education as terminal degree for many fields and toward articulation between community-college based programs in all fields and those in 4-year colleges and universities. Further, with the evolutionary changes predicted for health care delivery in the near future, the profession of nursing needs to provide its practitioners with the educational preparation necessary to meet the challenges of changing roles and delivery systems. The profession can achieve its goal of the BSN as entry to professional practice (Deback & Mentkowski, 1986; Primm, 1986; Young, Lehrer, & White, 1991). The RN/ BSN graduate can achieve the levels of knowledge, skill, and professional socialization desired by the profession and espoused by BSN program philosophies. Educators have determined valid measures for assessing prior knowledge and skill of RNs seeking the BSN degree, and have designed curricula that reflect adult learning theory and acknowledge the competing demands of work and personal life of the RN through alternate site instruction, flexible scheduling, and provision of a variety of support services. The confidence with which these statements can be made, however, will depend on the replication of studies reported in this review, and on the conduct of studies designed to assure generalizability of the results.

In spite of the commitment to baccalaureate education for entry positions in nursing practice, the majority of its practitioners are prepared in associate degree and diploma nursing programs. It would be interesting to have empirical evidence about the validity of a pattern the authors have observed in their practice. For economic and personal reasons many prospective RNs intentionally enroll in an ADN or diploma program while simultaneously seeking academic counseling about second-step program options. Their goal is to complete the general education requirements for the BSN level while in a prelicensure program. Of their own volition and with encouragement or mandates from employers, these graduates are seeking the baccalaureate degree in greater percentage than ever before. It is imperative, therefore, that processes be in place for the effective assessment of previous knowledge and skill, and for the efficient progression of the RN to degree completion.

ACKNOWLEDGMENT

Acknowledgment for assistance with search processes and materials retrieval is given to Mrs. Sue Ellen Ronk at Ashland University, and Ms. Cynthia Mathews and Mr. Rob Clay at The Ohio State University.

REFERENCES

Allen, C., Higgs, Z., & Holloway, J. (1988). Identifying students at risk for academic difficulty. *Journal of Professional Nursing, 4*, 113–118.

Baj, P. A. (1983). Stress of the returning R.N. student. In Holzemer, W. L., *Review of Research in Nursing Education* (pp. 92–106). Thorofare, NJ: Slack.

Baj, P. A. (1985). Demographic characteristics of RN and generic students: Implications for curriculum. *Journal of Nursing Education, 24*, 230–236.

Baker, S. S., & Barlow, D. J. (1988). Successful registered nurse education: A case analysis. *Nurse Educator, 13*(1), 18–22.

Banks, M. H. (1983). Validation of the General Health Questionnaire in a young community sample. *Psychological Medicine, 13*, 349–353.

Beck, D. L., & Srivastava, R. (1991). Perceived level and sources of stress in baccalaureate nursing students. *Journal of Nursing Education, 30*, 127–133.

Beeman, P. (1988). RNs' perceptions of their baccalaureate programs: Meeting their adult learning needs. *Journal of Nursing Education, 27*, 364–370.

Beeman, P. (1990). RN students in baccalaureate programs: Faculty's role and responsibility. *Journal of Continuing Education in Nursing, 21*(1), 42–45.

Boshier, R. (1973). Educational participation and dropout: A theoretical model. *Adult Education 23*(4), 132–135.

Boyd, R., & Apps, J. (1980). *Refining the discipline of adult education*. San Francisco, CA; Jossey-Bass.

Brooks, K. L., & Shepherd, J. M. (1992). Professionalism versus general thinking abilities of senior nursing students in four types of nursing curricula. *Journal of Professional Nursing, 8*(2), 87–95.

Chornick, N. L. (1992). A comparison of RN to BSN completion graduates to generic BSN graduates: Is there a difference? *Journal of Nursing Education, 31*, 203–209.

Cohen, J. B. (1967). An interpersonal orientation to the study of consumer behavior. *Journal of Marketing Research, 4*, 270–278.

Corwin, R. G. (1961). Role conception and career aspiration: A study of identity in nursing. *Social Quarterly, 2*, 69–86.

DeBack, V., & Mentkowski, M. (1986). Does the baccalaureate make a difference?: Differentiating nurse performance by education and experience. *Journal of Nursing Education, 25*, 275–285.

Deleruyelle, L., & Chally, P. (1984). Credit where credit is due. *American Journal of Nursing, 84*(1), 105–106.

Derstine, J. B. (1988). Anxiety in the adult learner in an RN to BSN program: Real or imagined. *Health Education, 19*(4), 13–15.

Dick, M., & Anderson, S. (1993). Job burnout in RN to BSN students: Relationships to life stress, time commitments and support for returning to school. *Journal of Continuing Education in Nursing, 24*(3), 105–109.

Firth, J. (1986). Level and sources of stress in medical students. *British Medical Journal, 292*, 1177–1180.

Firth, J., & Morrison, L. A. (1985). *The descriptions and reliabilities of coding systems for investigating stress in health professionals*. (MRC/ESRC SAPU Memo No. 757) University of Sheffield, England.

Fitts, W. H. (1965). *Manual: Tennessee self-concept scale*. Nashville, TN: Counselor Recordings and Tests.

Folkman, S., & Lazarus, R. (1985). If it changes, it must be progress: Study of emotion and coping during three stages of a college examination. *Journal of Personality and Social Psychology, 48*, 150–170.

Fotos, J. C. (1987). Characteristics of RN students continuing their education in a BS program. *Journal of Continuing Education in Nursing, 18*(4), 118–122.

Frances, K. T., & Naftel, D. L. (1983). Perceived sources of stress and coping strategies in allied health students: A model. *Journal of Allied Health, 12*, 262–272.

Garvey, J. (1983). An alternative baccalaureate curriculum plan for RNs. *Journal of Nursing Education, 22*, 216–219.

Goldberg, D. P. (1972). *The detection of Psychiatric Illness by Questionnaire.* London: Oxford University Press.

Gough, H. G. (1957). *The California Psychological Inventory.* Palo Alto, CA: Consulting Psychologists Press.

Guglielmino, L. M. (1980). *Norms and conversion table for Guglielmino's self-directed learning reading scale.* Unpublished manuscript.

Heinrich, K. T. & Gladstone, C. (1992). Orientation programs for nurse-adult learners: Fostering a sense of community. *Nurse Educator, 17*(1), 8–11.

Holmes, T. H., & Rahe, R. H. (1967). The social readjustment rating scale. *Journal of Psychosomatic Research, 11*, 213–218.

Holzemer, W. L. (Ed.) (1983). *Review of Research in Nursing Education.* New York: National League for Nursing.

Hughes, O., Wade, B., & Peters, M. (1991). The effects of a synthesis of nursing practice course on senior nursing students' self-concept and role perception. *Journal of Nursing Education, 30*, 69–72.

Kearney, R. T. (1991). Validation of prior nursing knowledge and performance in BSN education by RN students. *Journal of Nursing Education, 30*, 297–302.

King, J. E. (1986). A comparative study of adult developmental patterns of RN and generic students in a baccalaureate nursing program. *Journal of Nursing Education, 25*, 366–371.

King, J. E. (1988). Differences between RN and generic students and the impact of the educational process. *Journal of Nursing Education, 27*, 131–135.

Kolb, D. (1974). *Building a learning community.* Washington, DC: National Training and Development Service Press.

Kroll, C. (1990). Registered nurse students: Academic admission and progression. *Journal of Continuing Education in Nursing, 21*(4), 160–164.

Krouse, H. J. (1988). Personality characteristics of registered nurses in baccalaureate education. *Nurse Educator, 13*(5), 27, 36, 39.

Lange, L. L. (1986). Recruiting, advising, and program planning for RN/BSN students. *Western Journal of Nursing Research, 8*, 414–430.

Lawler, T. G., & Rose, M. A. (1987). Professionalization: A comparison among generic baccalaureate, ADN and RN/BN nurses. *Nurse Educator, 12*(3), 19–22.

Lee, E. J. (1987). Analysis of stressful clinical and didactic incidents reported by returning registered nurses. *Journal of Nursing Education, 26*, 372–379.

Lee, E. J. (1988). Analysis of coping methods reported by returning RNs. *Journal of Nursing Education, 27*, 309–313.

Linares, A. Z. (1989). A comparative study of learning characteristics of RN and generic students. *Journal of Nursing Education, 28*, 354–360.

Loevinger, J., & Wessler, R. (1970). *Measuring ego development: Construction and use of a sentence completion test.* San Francisco: Jossey-Bass.

Long, M. C., & Redding, B. A. (1991). Evaluating clinical skills of RN students. *Nurse Educator, 16*(3), 31–33.

Lynn, M. R., McCain, N. L., & Boss, B. J. (1991). Socialization of RN to BSN. *Image, 21*(4), 232–237.

Maslach, C., & Jackson, S. E. (1986). *Maslach burnout inventory manual* (2nd ed.) Palo Alto, CA: Consulting Psychologists Press.

Mattson, S. (1990). Coping and developmental maturity of R.N. baccalaureate students. *Western Journal of Nursing Research, 12*(4), 514–524.

McClelland, E., & Daly, J. (1991). A comparison of selected demographic character- istics and academic performance of on-campus and satellite-center RNs: Impli- cations for the curriculum. *Journal of Nursing Education, 30,* 261–266.

McHugh, M. K. (1991). Direct articulation of AD nursing students into an RN to BSN completion program: A research study. *Journal of Nursing Education, 30,* 293–296.

Megaree, E. I. (1972). *The California Psychological Inventory Handbook.* San Fran- cisco: Jossey-Bass.

Nowicki, S. Jr., & Duke, M. P. (1974). A locus of control scale for non-college as well as college adults. *Journal of Personality Assessment, 38,* 136–137.

O'Connor, A. (1979). Reasons nurses participate in continuing education. *Nursing Research, 31,* 354–359.

Oechsle, L., Volden, C., & Lambeth, S. (1990). Portfolios and RNs: An evaluation. *Journal of Nursing Education 29*(2), 54–59.

Periard, M. E., Bell, E. A., Knecht, L., & Woodman, E. A. (1991). Measuring effec- tive factors in RN/BSN programs. *Nurse Educator, 19*(6), 14–17.

Petrone, F. R. (1977). Challenging the challenge examinations. *Journal of Continuing Education in Nursing 10,* 23–29.

Primm, P. L. (1986). Entry into practice: Competency statements for BSNs and ADNs. *Nursing Outlook 34*(3), 135–137.

Rapson, M. F., Perry, L. A., & Parker, B. (1990). The relationship between selected educational outcomes of senior RN-to-BSN students and their choice of advanced placement options available in the Maryland nursing articulation model. *Journal of Professional Nursing 6*(2), 113–120.

Rawlins, T., Riordan, J., Delamaide, G., & Kilian, G. (1991). Student nurse recruit- ment: Determinants for choosing a nursing program. *Journal of Nursing Educa- tion 30*(5), 197–201.

Rendon, D. (1988) The registered nurse student: A role congruence perspective. *Jour- nal of Nursing Education 27,* 172–177.

Rezler, A. G., & Rezmovic, V. (1981). The learning preference inventory. *Journal of Allied Health, 10,* 28–34.

Rice, C. P. (1992). Strategies and faculty roles for teaching RN students. *Nurse Edu- cator 17*(1), 33–37.

Rose, M. A. (1988). ADN vs. BSN: The search for differentiation. *Nursing Outlook, 36*(6), 275–279.

Schwirian, P. M. (1985). Research on nursing students. In H. W. Wesley, & J. F. Fitzpatrick (Eds.), *Annual Review of Nursing Research* (vol. 2, pp. 211–237). New York: Springer Publishing Co.

Shepard, J. M., & Brooks, K. L. (1991). Self-concept among senior students in four types of nursing education programs. *Nurse Educator 16*(4), 8–9.

Slater-Stewart, D. (1979). Stewart Evaluation of Nursing Scale. Detroit: Wayne State University.

Spielberger, C. D., Gorsuch, R. L., Lushene, R., Vagg, P. R., & Jacobs, G. A. (1983). *Manual for the state-trait anxiety inventory.* Palo Alto, CA: Consulting Psychologists Press, Inc.

Stone, H., & Knopke, H. (1978). *Data gathering instruments for evaluating educational programs in the health sciences.* Madison, WI: University of Wisconsin.

Sullivan, E. J. (1987). Critical thinking, creativity, clinical performance, and achievement in RN students. *Nurse Educator, 12*(2), 12–16.

Throwe, A. N, & Fought, S. G. (1987). Landmarks in the socialization process from RN to BSN. *Nurse Educator 12*(6), 15–18.

Thurber, F. (1988). A comparison of RN students in two types of baccalaureate completion programs. *Journal of Nursing Education, 27,* 266–273.

Topf, M., & Dillon, E. (1988). Noise-induced stress as a predictor of burnout in critical care nurses. *Heart & Lung, 17,* 567–574.

Torrance, E. P. (1974). Torrance Tests of Creative Thinking: norms technical manual. Bensenville, IL: Scholastic Testing Service.

Viverais-Dresler, G., & Kutschke, M. (1992). RN students' satisfaction with clinical teaching in a distance education program. *Journal of Continuing Education in Nursing 23*(5), 224–230.

Wandelt, M. A. (1975). *Slater Nursing Competencies Rating Scale.* New York: Appleton-Century-Crofts.

Wang, A. M. (1991). Stressful and satisfying experiences of adult RN/BSN learners. *Nurse Educator 16*(5), 35–36.

Watson, A. B. (1983). Professional socialization of the registered nurse. In W. L. Hozemer, (Ed.), *Review of Research in Nursing Education* (pp. 34–59). Thorofare, NJ: Slack.

Watson, G., & Glaser, E. (1964). *Watson-Glaser Critical Thinking Appraisal Manual.* New York: Harcourt, Brace World.

Weathersby, R. (1977). A developmental perspective on adults' use of formal education (Doctoral dissertation, Harvard University). *Dissertation Abstracts International,* 38A, 7085A-7086A (University Microfilms No. 7808621).

Whelan, E. G. (1984). Role-orientation change among RNs in an upper division level baccalaureate program. *Journal of Nursing Education, 3,* 151–155.

Winston, R., Miller, T., & Prince, J. (1979). *Assessing student development.* Athens, GA: Student Development Associates.

Witt, B. S. (1992). The liberating effects of RN-to-BSN education. *Journal of Nursing Education 31,* 149–157.

Yang, J. C., & Noble, J. (1990). The validity of ACT-PEP test scores for predicting academic performance of registered nurses in BSN programs. *Journal of Professional Nursing 6*(6): 334–340.

Young, W. B., Lehrer, E. L., White, W. D. (1991). The effect of education on the practice of nursing. *Image, 23*(2), 105–108.

PART IV

Research on the
Profession of Nursing

Chapter 8

Minorities in Nursing

Diana L. Morris
Frances Payne Bolton School of Nursing
Case Western Reserve University

May L. Wykle
Frances Payne Bolton School of Nursing
Case Western Reserve University

CONTENTS

Minority participation in the nursing profession has been inextricably bound to the history of racism, segregation, and civil rights in the United States. Minority nurses continue to be underrepresented in spite of recent gains in the number of minority students enrolled in undergraduate nursing programs (Powell, 1992). The subpopulations with recognized minority status in the United States include blacks, Asian-Pacific Americans, Hispanics, and Native Americans. What little literature exists related to minorities in nursing is focused primarily on blacks, the largest minority group in nursing who are still underrepresented. Blacks comprise 12% of the population in the United States yet blacks represent 3.6% of all nurses and 4% of practicing nurses [American Nurses Association (ANA), 1988]. Further, the ANA reported that 89% of black nurses remain in active practice compared to 79% of white registered nurses. Asian-Pacific Americans represent 2% of registered nurses, Hispanic Americans 1.3%, and Native Americans 0.2%. Powell (1992) maintained that all minority nurses are more likely to remain active practitioners compared to white nurses.

For the purposes of this chapter, the following four ethnic minority categories were the focus of a literature search: blacks, Asian-Pacific, Hispanics, and Native Americans. Additional search category terms used were nursing, profession, and student. The Silver Platter 3.1 program was used for a MEDLINE Express search for pertinent citations from 1966 through July 1993; and the Cumulative Index of Nursing and Allied Health Literature (CINAHL) for 1983 through July 1993. The CINAHL indexes from 1960 through 1966 also were reviewed, adding the terms Negro and intergroup relations.

One citation was reported for the Asian and Hispanic classification, respectively using the terms: nursing and profession. One article addressed the educational and programmatic needs of Asian-Pacific students and the second article included discussion of recruitment of Hispanics to nursing. Two citations were identified for the Native American classification. One article focused on provision of health care to Native Americans rather than professional or educational development. The second citation contained a commentary on nursing practice in Houston, Texas that was published.

The majority of the citations were identified when either minority or black classifications were cross-referenced with nursing, profession, or student categories. In addition, bibliographic references from the search materials were reviewed for other pertinent citations. Twenty-one citations were related to historic and biographic topics. There were 47 citations that represented editorials, commentaries, and issue-driven materials. Citations that dealt with programmatic strategies and demonstration projects were identified regarding student recruitment and retention (28); clinical staff and administration (8); and professional advancement, particularly in academia (4). Ten citations provided information about student survival, professional development and research development opportunities, and contemporary minority nursing leaders. Nine empirical studies related to education of minority students, and two studies focused on professional nurses are reviewed in this chapter. Material from nonempirical citations are used in the chapter in order to broaden the discussion of the history and issues relevant to understanding the experience of minority nurses in the United States.

HISTORY

Citations of articles that had been published as early as 1902 were found. The citations included historic and biographic materials relative to black nurses as well as descriptions of early training programs for colored nurses. (The use of the term colored reflects normal language use in historic documents and period publications.) Mary Eliza Mahoney, recognized as the first trained black nurse, graduated in 1879 (Carnegie, 1991, 1992; Kalisch & Kalisch, 1986). She was admitted to a formal nurse training program at the New England Hospital for Women and Children to partially meet the quota for "one black and one Jew." Black men and women had functioned as nurses, however, particularly in times of war, prior to formalized training of nurses in this country (Carnegie, 1991; Hicks, 1990). For example, Mary Grant Seacole, a native of Jamaica, served with Nightingale in the Crimean War (Hicks, 1990). The rich history of blacks in nursing is well documented in the literature and reflects the struggle for racial equality in the United States (Campinha-Bacote, 1988; Carnegie, 1991; Hicks, 1990; Hine, 1985, 1989). Hine (1989) presented a history of black women in nursing from 1890 to 1950 within the context of racial conflict and cooperation.

Carnegie (1991) provided a history of blacks in nursing from 1854 through 1990. This history included material on key historic figures and contemporary nursing leaders. The evolution of segregated and later desegregated professional nursing organizations as well as access to professional practice in private, public, and military service settings were described. The development of black nursing students also was traced beginning with segregated education and quotas through the Cadet Nursing Program, the civil rights movement, desegregation, and the Breakthrough to Nursing program (Carnegie, 1986, 1988).

The first school of nursing for blacks was started in 1886 as a diploma program at Spelman College in Atlanta. The last black diploma program, Grady Hospital School of Nursing in Atlanta, closed in 1982 (Carnegie, 1991). The first baccalaureate nursing program exclusively for blacks was initiated at Howard University in 1922 (Carnegie, 1991). Prior to desegregation, such nursing programs for blacks provided nursing education opportunities to students who were prohibited from admission to all-white programs by segregation and exclusionary quota systems. These conditions existed throughout the country prior to the civil rights movement and affirmative action legislation of the 1960s. As expected, more programs designed exclusively for blacks existed in southern states than in the northern United States.

The Cadet Nurse Corps program was initiated in response to a critical nursing shortage during World War II. The 1943 Cadet Nurse Corps Act supported curriculum development and provided monies to predominantly black schools of nursing. As a result of the Cadet Nurse Corps program, access by black students to white schools of nursing was increased. Carnegie (1992) reported that at the time of the implementation of the Cadet Corps legislation, only 12 white schools admitted black students. This number was increased to 41 schools as a result of the Cadet program.

The Breakthrough to Nursing Project was developed in 1963, by the National Student Nurses' Association (NSNA), to recruit minorities into nursing (Carnegie, 1986). The project targeted blacks, Native Americans, Hispanics, and men in order to promote career opportunities in nursing and encourage nursing education programs to be more responsive to minority students' needs. The program received federal funding from 1966 through 1977. Such government support for minority group access to health professions was a result of civil rights activities.

The history of minority access to the profession was also addressed in a landmark program, Open Doors Wide in Nursing (ODWIN), initiated in 1964 by the Boston University School of Nursing Alumni (BUSON). Chaired by Mary Malone, the program enhanced minority access to nursing education (Scheinfeldt, 1967). ODWIN was designed to reach into the community through junior and senior high schools and organizations such as the Educational Counseling Committee of the Boston chapter of the National Association for the Advancement of Colored Persons (NAACP). BUSON Faculty and Alumni recognized that most young black women interested in nursing were counseled into licensed practical nursing schools and hospital diploma programs rather than baccalaureate programs. The purpose of the ODWIN project was to (a) acquaint young black women with nursing, (b) welcome them to the nursing profession, and (c) help them to succeed in nursing education programs. ODWIN received funding from the Sealantic and Kellogg Foundations. In addition to providing Future Nurses Clubs and supplemental classwork for high school students, supportive counseling was made available to students who had matriculated in a school of nursing. The Sealantic and Kellogg Foundations also funded nine additional ODWIN projects based on the Boston University model (Carnegie, 1991). With the development of the Breakthrough and ODWIN programs, Dr. Elizabeth Carnegie (1964) urged that the best of the white and black nursing schools openly recruit and admit students of all races.

The Kalisch and Kalisch (1986) history of American nursing provided an overview of the history of blacks in nursing, and the authors discussed the integration of black nurses into health care settings following the *Brown versus Board of Education of Topeka* Supreme Court decision. Additionally, the authors described the history of the only school of nursing established for Native Americans. Located in northeastern Arizona, the school operated from 1930 through the mid-1950s (Kalisch & Kalisch, 1986). The school enrolled Native American women from 12 states and approximately 25 tribes. Students practiced in the school's parent hospital, which provided services largely to members of the Navajo Nation. It is interesting to note that the Association of American Indian (Native American) Nurses group, which has struggled to exist and was listed as an active organization by the ANA in 1992, was not mentioned in the Kalisch and Kalisch discussion of minorities in nursing. Also not noted in the Kalisch and Kalisch history of American nursing was the National Association of Hispanic Nurses (NAHN) created in the late 1970s and currently with 20 active chapters in the United States. The Association's goals are focused on health care services for Hispanics and the advancement of Hispanic nurses (NAHN, 1993).

The history of black nurses' struggle to be full participants in professional organizations epitomizes experiences of all minority nurses in the United States. At the inception of the ANA, black nurses were excluded from membership. As early as 1879, black graduate nurses were beginning to organize themselves. In 1908, 52 black nurses met in New York City to formalize the organization of the National Association of Colored Graduate Nurses (NACGN) (Campinha-Bacote, 1988; Carnegie, 1991). It was not until the period of 1949 to 1951 that NACGN and ANA worked toward dissolution of NACGN and integration of black nurses into the ANA. Leadership for this historic move was spearheaded by Mabel Staupers, a nurse of Irish and black heritage, who had been an executive of NACGN and was elected president of ANA in 1949 (Campinha-Bacote, 1988). In 1970, however, black nurses met at the ANA convention to discuss their concerns about the professional advancement of black nurses, health care needs of the black community, and a lack of attention to minority concerns within ANA. Dr. Lauranne Sams organized a meeting of black nurses at the home of Dr. Mary Harper in Cleveland, Ohio, and the National Black Nurses Association (NBNA) came into being (Carnegie, 1991). The NBNA continues to support access to nursing education and professional advancement for black nurses as well as all minority nurses, and access to culturally competent health care for the black community and other underserved populations.

EDUCATION

The critical underrepresentation of minorities in the nursing profession raises concerns about minority enrollment in undergraduate nursing education, the pipeline for professional nursing. Thus discussions of minorities in nursing most often address recruitment and retention of students in education programs. In 1991 the American Association of Colleges of Nursing (AACN) reported that 9.9% of students enrolled in undergraduate programs were black Americans; 3% Hispanic Americans; 2.5% Asian Americans; and 0.5% Native Americans. In 1989 blacks accounted for 13.5% of the students enrolled in associate degree and diploma programs, according to the National League for Nursing (NLN) (1990). Rosenfeld (1991) reported that minorities accounted for 18% of the admissions to schools of nursing in 1990. Black Americans represented 11.1% of admissions to schools of nursing, Hispanic Americans 3.2%, Asian Americans 3%, and Native Americans 0.6%. Even more striking is the underrepresentation of minority nurses enrolled in master's degree programs. AACN (1991) reported that blacks represented only 6% of master's programs enrollment with 2.3% Asian, 1.8% Hispanic, and 0.4% Native American. Blacks were the largest minority group matriculated in doctoral programs but account for only 4% of the total enrollment (AACN, 1991). Carnegie (1992) reported that there were approximately 200 black nurses with earned doctorates in the United States, a considerable increase in the last 10 years.

An example of early research that was focused on minority nursing students was a 1961 study published in *Nursing Research*. Redden and Scales (1961) examined the effect of nursing education on 15 personality characteristics in a sample of 104 nursing students at a historically black college. The longitudinal study included data collected at the beginning of the freshman year, the end of the sophomore year, and the spring semester of the senior year. The Edwards Personal Preference schedule was used to examine manifest needs such as autonomy, aggression, and deference, which were purported to be personality variables. At the beginning of the freshman year, the black female nursing students were compared to a normative group of college women of unstated minority and nonminority status. The black nursing students had significantly different scores from the normative sample on 12 of the 15 personality characteristics at time one of the data collection. This comparison seems to have been done for descriptive purposes only. When baseline data were collected at the beginning of the freshman year were compared with senior-year data, only 2 of the 15 characteristics were significantly different. By the senior year of the education program, only two of the 15 characteristics were significantly different (order, abasement) within the black student sample. Based on these findings, the authors suggested that the nursing education process had little effect on changes in black students' personality characteristics. What characteristics one may or may not want to change as a result of nursing education and the significance of these characteristics to the development of minority students were unclear. Although early study focused on change within the student, the major foci of the literature on minority nursing students has been on recruitment and retention.

Powell (1992) estimated that one-third of the black students enrolled in undergraduate programs do not graduate. Historic black colleges and universities account for approximately one quarter (23%) of black nursing graduates (Powell, 1992), even though these institutions account for only 2% of baccalaureate enrollment in the United States (AACN, 1992). The significance of recruitment and retention issues with minority students is twofold. First, although enrollment of minorities, specifically blacks, has increased, student attrition has continued to be remarkably high (Allen, Nunley, & Scott-Warner, 1988; Buckley, 1980; Jones, 1992; Powell, 1992; Rodgers, 1990; Tucker-Allen, 1989). Second, the pool of potential undergraduate students, and thus potential nursing students, reflects the growth of minority populations in the United States (Andrews, 1992; Farrell, 1988). Much of the literature personifies application of knowledge that addresses the educational and academic support needs of minority students in undergraduate nursing programs at predominantly white institutions. For example, one author (Crow, 1993) described the use of a "Native American World View" when working with Native American nursing students and compared this perspective to the "Nursing Academic View." Additionally, Davis (1992) discussed African theory in relation to contemporary minority students.

Stevens and Walker (1993) surveyed 641 college-bound high school seniors in metropolitan Washington, DC, to determine why nursing was or was not selected as a career. For this descriptive cross-sectional study, the researchers used a convenience sample from both private and public institutions. Descriptive statistics were used to examine decisions to choose or not to choose nursing. Students who choose nursing as a career were significantly more likely to be black females between the ages of 16 and 17. Those students who said they would choose nursing as a career had past experiences with nurses or illness and perceived certain characteristics of the nursing profession to be positive, such as helping others. Of the sample 97.3% did not choose nursing as a career, however. The sample for this study was not representative of high school students but only those students who were declared to be college bound. Students who have an interest in a nursing career and the potential to be nursing students, or students who have been counseled to attend noncollegiate programs such as practical nursing, diploma, or associate-degree programs would be excluded. The "college-bound" inclusion criteria are of particular concern when the possibility exists that minority students may be less likely to be counseled into college-bound programs in some school systems. A longitudinal, correlation study using a representative sample that follows minority students after high school graduation to determine actual career choice, could be helpful in the development of a predictive model for identifying prospective students.

Other researchers examined the effectiveness of two education support programs to increase the likelihood of success among undergraduate students. In one study researchers evaluated a prematriculation summer program for minority students at the Medical College of Georgia School of Nursing in 1985 (Cook & Thurmand, 1988/1989). The focus was on programmatic evaluation of a prematriculation program and did not examine student success post matriculation. An evaluation study by Goodman, Blake, and Lott (1990) examined the effectiveness of a computer-assisted instruction (CAI) program to support classroom instruction and peer tutoring by comparing unit tests and NLN exams in medical-surgical nursing. Scores were compared for two different groups of students during two consecutive academic years. Higher scores resulted when the CAI was instituted but it is unclear as to whether tests of significance were used.

Allen, Nunley, and Scott-Warner (1988) examined factors that influence admission and retention of black nursing students in predominantly white institutions and black institutions. A convenience sample included students, faculty, and administrators from one public and one private institution in four regions of the United States. The study, completed in 1984, reported differences in students', black faculty's, and white faculty's ratings on barriers to admission and retention. The data were compared to ratings from a study of black students, and black and white faculty in seven predominantly white universities (Smith, 1980) using the same design and questionnaire. Although barriers to recruitment and retention were identified, comparison between groups in the sample was limited to percentage of subjects who perceive a particular item as important. It would be helpful to design a longitudinal study using a representative sample to determine, particularly for students, if perceptions of barriers can predict retention and academic success. One could also examine congruence between student and faculty perceptions and variables related to recruitment and retention. More important, 10 years have passed since the study, with a great deal of political and economic change. In addition, the characteristics and expectations of persons enrolling in undergraduate nursing programs have changed and now include a cohort of younger blacks and an older black cohort, beginning or changing careers.

The results of three correlation studies in which researchers examined predictors of success in minority students also should be viewed with caution given the passage of time. Generalizability of each study is limited because each was done within a specific institution. Outtz (1979) studied predictors of success on the State Board Test Pool Examination (SBTPE) for a sample of 110 black nursing students who graduated from a public university between 1971 and 1973. Independent variables included high school grade point average (GPA); college GPAs; high school and college science courses GPA; and scores on the Scholastic Achievement Test (SAT). The researcher reported that the cumulative college GPA was the best predictor of success on the SBTPE, followed by verbal SAT scores.

Using discriminant analysis, Dell and Halpin (1984) examined predictors of graduation in a predominately black undergraduate program and predictors of success on state board examinations using student data from 1970 through 1974. Thus, the study was carried out prior to the current national state board examination procedure. Dell and Halpin found that high school GPA, SAT scores, and scores on the NLN Pre-Nursing Examination significantly differentiated between graduates and students who left the program. Success on SBTPE was best predicted by college GPA, followed by SAT verbal scores and NLN Pre-Test scores.

In the second study researchers used student data from black students ($n = 111$) and an aggregate of Asian-Pacific, Hispanic, and Native American students ($n = 34$) attending a predominantly white state university (Boyle, 1986). The subgroup of Asian-Pacific, Hispanic, and Native American students was so small that it was not possible to analyze results from these groups separately, however. The students had attended the university from 1971 through 1981 so that both SBTPE scores and National Comprehensive Licensure Examination of Registered Nurses (NCLEX-RN) scores were used. In the Boyle study, entering grade point average (ENGPA) and the American College Test Assessment (ACT) were the best predictors of success on state board exams. Less variance was explained by ENGPA and ACT with the black students.

It is difficult to compare the findings of these three studies because the same variables were not used. For example, Dell and Halpin (1984) included scores on the NLN Pre-Nursing Examination, Outtz (1979) and Boyle (1986) did not. Additionally, although each of the researchers included GPA as a variable, Outtz used cumulative college GPA, Dell and Halpin used high school GPA, and Boyle selected ENGPA. Although not entirely clear, it seemed that Boyle's variable ENGPA was GPA on matriculation to the nursing school, which could be students' GPAs during prenursing liberal arts study. More current and rigorous research knowledge is needed to better inform nursing educators and the profession about variables that predict contemporary minority student success. Studies should be conducted to examine both the dependent variables addressed in these studies: retention through graduation and success on state board examinations. A representative sample with a longitudinal design that consistently includes variables such as GPA and required achievement tests used in nursing education programs would be valuable and helpful.

Two studies were identified in which the researchers evaluated the effectiveness of programs designed to support minority students in baccalaureate and graduate programs. Drice, Hunter, and Williams (1978) examined the effects of utilization of academic support programs on improved GPA at graduation for Asian-Pacific ($n = 12$), black ($n = 22$), and Chicano ($n = 4$) students between 1971 through 1979 at a public university. The authors reported that both the Asian-Pacific and black students had significantly higher GPAs at graduation. Interestingly the authors reported both users and nonusers of the tutorial programs had significantly increased GPAs at graduation. The small numbers of different minority students used in the study limit the value of any study results and interpretations. The fact that both users and nonusers of the tutorial programs had higher GPAs, suggests that the independent variable may be the total education program. Another program evaluation study was conducted by Memmer and Worth (1991) to examine retention of English-as-a-Second-Language (ESL) students. Data were obtained for 21 generic undergraduate nursing programs regarding the types and numbers of retention approaches used at each institution. The number of ELS students in the 21 nursing programs ranged from 6% to 24% of the respective program's total enrollment. Nonparametric analysis suggested that the programs with the highest retention rates of ELS students used a greater number of the 47 retention approaches reported by the 21 programs. The actual demographic characteristics of the ELS students attending the 21 programs were not reported. It would be particularly meaningful to develop systematic knowledge that clearly identifies the critical characteristics of retention programs, which in fact support the outcome of increased retention of minority students in collegiate nursing programs.

Eyres, Loustau, and Ersek (1992) examined ways of knowing among beginning nursing students. A phenomenological design was used that included a semistructured questionnaire suggested by Balance, Clinch, Goldberger, and Tarule (1986). A convenience sample of 21 first-quarter nursing students at a university-affiliated program included 16 women and five men. Only minority women were included in the sample, three of whom used English as a second language and may have been immigrants though it was unclear. The researchers reported that the minority students' responses were more indicative of received knowers and related these results to the students' cultural background. Such a conclusion is difficult to evaluate because the students' specific minority group membership is not addressed. The validity of any results and interpretations is questionable given the small number of students, even for this type of design, and the possibility that some of the minority students may be immigrants to the United States. The purpose of the study, to examine ways of knowing in beginning students, has merit. In order to be useful to nurse educators, however, broad-based systematic inquiry that includes representative samples with adequate numbers of minority students is necessary. One also needs to consider the potential differences between racial/ethnic minority students who are lifetime residents of the United States and those persons who may be assigned racial minority membership but are immigrants to the United States. In addition, diversity within minority groups also needs to be examined.

PROFESSIONAL DEVELOPMENT

There is a dearth of systematic research on the success and professional development of minority nurses. Historical reviews (Carnegie, 1991; Hine, 1985, 1989) have chronicled the often barrier-laden career trajectories of black nurses. Anecdotally, it has been pointed out that black nurses often need to have acquired higher degrees and that it takes a longer period of time for black nurses to obtain promotions. This also is likely to be the experience of nurses from other ethnic minority groups.

Carnegie (1991) reported that the majority of black nursing leaders admitted to the American Academy of Nursing had at least a portion of their educational experiences in one of the predominantly black colleges and/or universities. Nursing leaders have written about the need for mentor-protegé relationships as a component of affirmative action (Weekes, 1989). In one doctoral dissertation the researcher compared the behaviors of black and white nursing leaders (Yearwood, 1983). Other authors have provided information regarding postdoctoral leadership development (Bessent, 1989) and research training (Harden, 1992). In editorials and position papers black nurses, as well as other minorities, are challenged to prepare themselves for academic and clinical leadership (Doswell, 1988/1989; Harper, 1987/1988; Hussein, 1989; Powell, 1991). Giger, Johnson, Davidhizar, and Fishman (1993) recently addressed the need to develop strategies for building representative nursing faculties. The challenge to minority nurses to pursue advance education is related by authors to the critical health care needs of minority groups, the lack of substantive minority research, and the paucity of doctorally prepared minority faculty.

There are a few empirical studies that address practice and professional development of the clinician. For example, Schmieding (1991) described a program at a large teaching hospital to retain minority nurses and their professional advancement. The program and its implementation are described, but no systematic evaluation of outcomes is reported. Another author briefly addressed the stresses black nurses experience in the work environment and stress management techniques were suggested (Banks, 1986). Again no systematic inquiry was reported to provide data on stresses unique to black nurses in a particular organization, nor was the efficacy of stress management interventions examined.

Greener, Paine, LeeDecher, and Gray (1989) reported results of a cross-sectional survey of nurse-midwives to obtain needs-assessment data regarding the organization of and services provided by American College of Nurse Midwives (ACNM). Questionnaires were sent to a mailing list of certified nurse-midwives, both members and nonmembers, with a 39.4% response rate. Minority nurse-midwives who responded included blacks, Asian-Pacifics, Hispanics, Native Americans, and unidentified "others," and represented 4.3% ($n = 74$) of the sample. For analysis, all minority subjects were grouped as nonwhite. Cross-tabulations indicated some significant differences between white and nonwhite groups for specific variables. Nonwhites were less likely to be members; had less confidence in elected officers; were more likely to say that ACNM did not address current professional issues well; valued membership in ACNM less; and rated ACNM's communication as poorer. The small number of minority respondents made it impossible to discern differences between and within minority groups or between particular minority groups and the white group. Also, one category included in the nonwhite group was "other" but no information was provided to describe responses to this category.

An early study of minority nurses in clinical institutions was reported by Goldstein (1960), a sociologist. The study was done from 1951 to 1952 to examine integration of black nurses into hospital settings in the Midwest. The design was seemingly ethnographic in nature using informants, including 23 black nurses, and personal observations by the researcher. Three hospital settings were used: a Jewish hospital, a university hospital, and a black hospital. The nature of each hospital's organizational culture and the role of minority nurses greatly influenced black nurses' experiences. If the hospital began to integrate staff as a result of the World War II nursing shortage with a spirit of resignation rather than commitment to integration, blacks were usually not supported in the role of nurse and left to deal with discrimination by themselves. The study was an attempt to identify organizational behaviors that supported the role of the black nurse in hospitals. The need to systematically examine organizational cultures in which minority practitioners and faculty function is relevant today. Malone (1993) has suggested strategies for support of culturally diverse care provided by a culturally diverse staff that can be implemented by nursing administrators in clinical settings. Also, Giger and colleagues (1993) recently proposed strategies for developing representative nursing faculties. Outcome evaluation of such strategies could provide meaningful information for clinical and academic nursing administrators in order to provide access and career opportunities to minority nurses. We have not as yet developed empirical knowledge that can guide the profession in supporting the development and advancement of minority nurses in existing practice and academic settings.

FUTURE DIRECTIONS

There is a dire need for systematic investigation of strategies for recruitment, retention, and professional development of minority nurses. Considering past history and the continued underrepresentation of minorities in undergraduate and graduate nursing programs and losses due to attrition, empirical knowledge is needed to guide programming for recruitment and retention of students and development of minority faculty. Studies are needed to identify predictors of minority student success in contemporary student groups and professional advancement of minority nurses and that also identify within-group differences. The current categorization of ethnic minority group status ignores the diversity within minority groups. Blacks, Asian-Pacifics, Hispanics, and Native Americans are not homogeneous groups. In fact within-group differences may be greater and have more influence than between-group differences. It is important to be clear that persons of color who have immigrated to the United States may have different characteristics and outcomes than native-born citizens of color. Variables addressing intragroup differences and immigration status need to be considered and incorporated into research models to obtain valid findings.

We need to move beyond program evaluation in both nursing education and professional development to outcome research that can provide empirical bases for the advancement and success of minority persons in educational and service organizations. There needs to be more systematic investigation of the influence of culturally competent faculty on the educational experiences of minority nursing students and minority nurses. Further study is required to determine the influence of minority nurses on the health care delivery system and the health care of persons of color.

As a new century is approaching, the discipline of nursing can look forward to embracing and celebrating the diversity within our profession and community. Systematic investigation, relative to the growing diversity of the potential candidate pool for professional nurses and subsequent professional advancement of culturally diverse nursing graduates to meet the needs of people served by nurses will require continuous development of pertinent empirical knowledge. Such inquiry will be necessary to inform the profession and support the evolution of the discipline.

REFERENCES

Allen, M. E., Nunley, J. C., & Scott-Warner, M. (1988). Recruitment and retention of black students in baccalaureate nursing programs. *Journal of Nursing Education*, *27*, 107–116.

American Association of Colleges of Nursing (1991). *1990–91, enrollment and graduations in baccalaureate and graduate programs in nursing*. Washington, DC: Author.

American Association of Colleges of Nursing. (1992). *Customized report on enrollment and graduations for historically black colleges and universities*. Washington, DC: Author.

American Nurses Association. (1988). *Facts about nursing*. Kansas City, MO: Author.

Andrews, M. M. (1992). Cultural perspectives on nursing in the 21st century. *Journal of Professional Nursing*, *8*, 7–15.

Balance, M. F., Clinch, B. M., Goldberger, N. R., & Tarule, J. M. (1986). *Women's ways of knowing: The development of self, voice, and mind*. New York: Basic Books.

Banks, J. (1986). Stress management for black nurses. *Journal of the National Black Nurses Association*, *1*(1), 61–65.

Bessent, H. (1989). Postdoctoral leadership training for women of color. *Journal of Professional Nursing*, *5*, 278–282.

Boyle, K. K. (1986). Predicting the success of minority students in a baccalaureate nursing program. *Journal of Nursing Education*, *25*, 186–192.

Buckley, J. (1980). Faculty commitment to retention and recruitment of black students. *Nursing Outlook*, *28*, 46–50.

Campinha-Bacote, J. (1988). The black nurses' struggle toward equality: An historical account of the national association of colored graduate nurses. *Journal of the National Black Nurses Association*, *2*(2), 15–25.

Carnegie, M. E. (1964). Are Negro schools of nursing needed today? *Nursing Outlook, 12*(2), 52–56.

Carnegie, M. E. (1986). *The paths we tread/blacks in nursing.* Philadelphia: Lippincott.

Carnegie, M. E. (1988). Breakthrough to nursing: Twenty five years of involvement. *Imprint, 35*(2), 55–56, 59.

Carnegie, M. E. (1991). *The path we tread: Blacks in nursing 1854–1990* (2nd ed.). New York: National League for Nursing Press.

Carnegie, M. E. (1992). Black nurses in the United States: 1879–1992. *Journal of the National Black Nurses Association, 6*(1), 13–18.

Cook, P. R., & Thurmand, V. (1988/1989). Summer program for pre-matriculating nursing students. *Journal of the National Black Nurses Association, 3*(1), 54–63.

Crow, K. (1993). Multiculturalism and pluralistic thought in nursing education: Native American world view and the nursing academic world view. *Journal of Nursing Education, 32,* 198–204.

Davis, S. P. (1992). Africanity theory and the new student in nursing. *Journal of Black Nursing Faculty, 3*(2), 26–30.

Dell, M. A., & Halpin, G. (1984). Predictors of success in nursing school and on state board examinations in a predominantly black baccalaureate nursing program. *Journal of Nursing Education, 23,* 147–150.

Doswell, W. M. (1988/1989). Nursing research needs of black Americans: 1989 and beyond. *Journal of the National Black Nurses Association, 3*(1), 45–53.

Drice, A. D , Hunter, V., & Williams, B. S. (1978). The influence of academic support programs on retention of minority nursing students: A descriptive study. *Journal of Nursing Education, 17*(3), 22–34.

Eyres, S. J., Loustau, A., & Ersek, M. (1992) Ways of knowing among beginning students of nursing. *Journal of Nursing Education, 31,* 175–180.

Farrell, J. (1988). The changing pool of candidates for nursing. *Journal of Professional Nursing, 4* 145, 230.

Giger, J. N., Johnson, J. Y., Davidhizar, R., & Fishman, D. (1993). Strategies for building a representative nursing faculty. *Nursing & Health Care, 14,* 144–150.

Goldstein, R. L. (1960). Negro nurses in hospital. *The American Journal of Nursing, 60,* 215–217.

Goodman, J., Blake, J., & Lott, M. (1990). CAI: A strategy for retaining minority and academically disadvantaged students. *Nurse Educator, 15*(2), 37–41.

Greener, D. L., Paine, L. L., LeeDecher, C. A., & Gray, C. A. (1989). Nurse-midwives speak out on the ACNM. *Journal of Nurse-Midwifery, 34,* 21–30.

Harden, J. T. (1992). National institutes of health extramural associates program: Research opportunity. *Journal of the Black Nurses Association, 5*(2), 45–53.

Harper, M. S. (1987/1988). Guest editorial: Research in nursing. *Journal of the National Black Nurses Association, 2*(1), 9–10.

Hicks, L. (1990). *A review of the literature and related research: A descriptive study of Black nurses, the challenge of needed change.* Unpublished doctoral dissertation. Wayne State University, Detroit, MI.

Hine, D. C. (Ed.). (1985). *Black women in the nursing profession: A documentary history.* New York: Garland.

Hine, D. C. (1989). *Black women in white: Racial conflict and cooperation in the nursing profession, 1890–1950.* Bloomington, IN: Indiana University Press.

Hussein, C. A. (1989). Black America year 2000: Challenges of tomorrow. *Journal of the National Black Nurses Association, 3*(2), 57–62.

Jones, S. H. (1992). Improving retention and graduation rates for black students in nursing education: A developmental model. *Nursing Outlook, 40*, 78–85.

Kalisch, P. A., & Kalisch, B. J. (1986). *The advance of American nursing*, (2nd ed.). Boston: Little, Brown

Malone, B. L. (1993). Caring for culturally diverse racial groups: An administrative matter. *Nursing Administrative Quarterly, 17*(2), 21–29.

Memmer, M. K., & Worth, C. C. (1991). Retention of english-as-a-second-language (ESL) students: Approaches used by California's 21 generic baccalaureate nursing programs. *Journal of Nursing Education, 30*, 389–396.

National Association of Hispanic Nurses. (1993). NAHN conference: Leading the way. *Minority Nurse Professional*, 60–61.

National League for Nursing. (1990). *Nursing student census. 1989*. Pub. No. 19–2291. New York: Author.

Outtz, J. H. (1979). Predicting the success on state board examinations for blacks. *Journal of Nursing Education, 18*(9), 35–40.

Powell, D. L. (1991). Health care crisis in the black community: Challenges prospects, and the black nurse. *Journal of the National Black Nurses Association, 5*(1), 3–9.

Powell, D. L. (1992). The recruitment and retention of African American nurses: An analysis of current data. *Journal of the National Black Nurses Association, 6*(1), 3–12.

Redden, J. W. & Scales, E. E. (1961). Nursing education and personality characteristics. *Nursing Research, 10*, 215–218.

Rodgers, S. G. (1990). Retention of minority nursing students on predominantly white campuses. *Nurse Educator, 15*(5), 36–39.

Rosenfeld, P. (1991). *Nursing datasource 1991: Volume I trends in contemporary nursing education*. Pub. No. 19–2420. New York: National League for Nursing.

Scheinfeldt, J. (1967). Opening doors wider in nursing. *American Journal of Nursing, 67*, 1461–1464.

Schmieding, N. J. (1991). A novel approach to recruitment, retention, and advancement of minority nurses in a health care organization. *Nursing Administration Quarterly, 15*(4), 69–76.

Smith, D. H. (1980). Admission and retention problems of black students at seven predominantly white universities. *National Advisory Committee on Black Higher Education*. Washington, DC: U.S. Department of Education.

Stevens, K. A., & Walker, E. A. (1993). Choosing a career; Why not nursing for more high school seniors? *Journal of Nursing Education, 32*, 13–17.

Tucker-Allen, S. (1989). Losses incurred through minority student nurse attrition. *Nursing & Health Care, 10*, 395–397.

Weekes, D. P. (1989). Mentor-protege relationships: A critical element in affirmative action. *Nursing Outlook, 37*, 156–157.

Yearwood, A. C. (1983). *Behaviors of black and white nursing leaders*. Unpublished doctoral dissertation. Columbia University Teacher's College, New York.

PART V

Other Research

Chapter 9

Native American Health

SHAROL F. JACOBSON
COLLEGE OF NURSING
UNIVERSITY OF OKLAHOMA HEALTH SCIENCES CENTER

CONTENTS

Methods of the Review

On almost every indicator of morbidity, mortality, and quality of life Native Americans (NAs) are substantially worse off than the dominant culture and as bad or worse off than other minorities (Heckler, 1985). Compared to the US population, over twice as many NAs are unemployed or live in poverty (Rhoades, Reyes, & Buzzard, 1987). Approximately 60% of NA students drop out of high school before twelfth grade (McShane, 1988). Although the death rate for NA infants is now approximately equal to that for all races (Rhoades, D'Angelo, & Hurlburt, 1987), postneonatal deaths and deaths from sudden infant death syndrome are nearly twice as common among NAs as in the general population [Indian Health Service (IHS), 1990]. The prevalence of diabetes among NAs exceeds 20% in many tribes and reaches 50% among two Arizona tribes [Department of Health and Human Services (DHHS), 1990]. The NA death rate from alcoholism is four times higher than the national average (Lamarine, 1988). Alcoholism is also related to an incidence of fetal alcohol syndrome six times greater than in the general population (Honigfeld & Kaplan, 1987), to over 60% of cases of child abuse and neglect (Lujan, DeBruyn, May, & Bird, 1989), to 75% of accidents (the second leading cause of death among NA men), and to a homicide rate 60% higher than that of the general population. The suicide rates among various NA tribes (also related to alcoholism) are three to 10 times the rates for the general population (DHHS, 1990).

Nurses represent a relatively untapped resource for research on NA health care. Nursing's emphasis on the holistic understanding of human experience and cultural perspectives as a precondition for effective health care is more consistent with traditional NA values than the biomedical perspective (Henderson & Primeaux, 1981). The Indian Health Service has acknowledged the unique perspective of nursing and called for increased emphasis on nursing research, particularly in relation to the control of chronic disease (Arnold, Koertvelyessy, Berg, & Nutting, 1989).

METHODS OF THE REVIEW

Definitions of Key Terms

Although differences of opinion about what to call the preColumbian peoples of North America are recognized, they are referred to here as Native Americans. This term subsumes Alaska Natives who do not wish to be known as American Indians. Persons or institutions of nonNA society will be referred to as Anglos, Western, or whites. Nursing research is defined broadly to include studies done by nurses as principal investigators or studies by nonnurses that include nurses as junior authors.

Search Strategies and Contents of the Review

Several strategies were used to locate relevant literature. In the invisible college approach, the reviewer contacted colleagues with research or service ties to NA health for articles or names of other investigators. The ancestry approach involved tracking citations from one study to another. The descendency approach involved retrieving citations from topical indexes manually and by computer and screening them for topic relevance. Indexes and collections used included MEDLINE, Cumulative Index of Nursing and Allied Health Literature (CINAHL), Psychological Abstracts, and the Western History Collection at the University of Oklahoma. A very broad range of keywords was used initially, including racial and cultural names for the population (American Indian, Alaska Native, Native American), combinations of racial and cultural names with health or healing terms (American Indian health, traditional medicine/healing), disciplinary or subdisciplinary headings (anthropology, transcultural nursing, nursing research, public health, racial and ethnic studies), and names of diseases or health problems of known importance in NA health (accidents, alcoholism, diabetes, and so on). The search terms were then narrowed to those found to locate relevant materials most efficiently, which were Native American, clinical research, nursing research, and the disease entities. Manual searches of indexes and journals were also performed to follow up on promising leads and capitalize on serendipity.

In this chapter all published studies located that were done by nurses as principal investigators or involved nurses as members of the research team since 1980 ($N = 29$) are reviewed. Errors of omission of nurse authors may have occurred because this cannot always be determined from the publication. The start date of 1980 (for all but a very few classic works) coincides with the start of a decade of major positive changes in the quantity and quality of nursing research (Stevenson, 1992) and with changes in morbidity profiles of NAs from mostly infectious to mostly chronic diseases (DHHS, 1990). Some Canadian studies are included, as native populations and health professionals in Canada face problems similar to those in the United States.

The review also includes some nonnursing studies considered to be of particular substantive or methodological interest to nurses. These articles met three or more of the following criteria: (a) representation of an important NA health problem, some aspect of which is or could be within the purview of nursing, (b) representation of common or new data-gathering techniques in research on NA health, (c) representation of a major author or research program on NA health, (d) work by an NA author, (e) attention to culture as an important factor in health needs and care, and (f) useful substantive or methodological guidance for future research.

The review does not include dissertations, research reports from *The IHS Primary Care Provider* (the newsletter of the Indian Health Service), or articles dealing solely with the physiology of NA disease or in which NAs were only incidentally included in the sample. Books about NA culture or health were not included unless they contained classic or especially timely work of nurse authors or other investigators. Because of the breadth of the topic of Native American health, gaps in the research literature are identified in individual sections of the review where they are most relevant for generalizations about the state of nursing research knowledge of NA health.

HISTORICAL, SOCIAL, AND POLITICAL CONTEXTS OF NATIVE AMERICAN HEALTH

The effective study of NA health requires that investigators go beneath the romanticized stereotypes of NA cultures to appreciate the historical, social, and political contexts of NA life and health. Although a full description is beyond the scope of this chapter, the following brief information is particularly relevant to the understanding and critique of research literature on NAs and the planning of new studies. The turbulent history of NA–US government relations, characterized by alternating periods of neglect and active intervention, has engendered a profound mistrust of nonnatives among many NAs. Investigators of NA child health, for example, will quickly realize that the historic placement of 25% to 40% of NA children in nonNA foster care or adoptive homes (McShane, 1988) hampers their acceptance by NAs. The civil rights activity of the 1960s affected NAs as well as other races and renewed an emphasis on pantribal alliances and councils and on Indian sovereignty in which tribes expect to be treated as independent nations (Brod & LaDue, 1989). The sovereignty issue in conjunction with extensively publicized research on such sensitive issues as alcohol and child abuse has provoked bitter charges of insensitivity and cultural imperialism against nonNA investigators and led to strict oversight of research procedures and publication by many NA tribes (Shore, 1989).

Although great strides were made in NA health when the Indian Health Service (IHS) was transferred from the Bureau of Indian Affairs to the Public Health Service in 1955, the IHS is no longer the only provider of health care to NAs. Increasingly, tribes and intertribal organizations operate their own hospitals and clinics or contract for health services (Rhoades et al., 1987). The July/August 1987 issue of *Public Health Reports* contains a special section entitled "Health Services for American Indians." This feature provides an authoritative, comprehensive description of the programs, accomplishments, and challenges of the Indian Health Service. Health care for NAs has also been complicated by the migration of over 54% of NAs to urban areas, where they encounter a dearth of IHS facilities, unaffordable care, and a reluctance of other providers to care for them because of uncertainties of reimbursement (Brod & LaDue, 1989).

Data about NAs are not comprehensive. Certain tribes (particularly from the Southwest) have been studied intensively, whereas others have received little research attention. The problems of urban NAs are much less studied than those of rural and reservation people. Population studies and longitudinal studies of NAs are rare. Because of a lack of a definition of the demographic and cultural characteristics of tribes in the available literature, the extensive negotiations needed to arrange for a random or stratified sample of people across tribes, and the highly uneven geographic distribution of NAs (Beauvais, Oetting, & Edwards, 1985), studies of NAs with representative samples are difficult to achieve, and most reports are based on convenience or clinical samples. Official data from the IHS, the US Census, and state offices of vital statistics are subject to underreporting of NA vital events and do not identify tribal backgrounds. Information on NAs is limited or even absent from such nationwide surveys as the Adult Use of Tobacco Survey, the National Health and Nutrition Examination Surveys (NHANES I and II), the National Health Interview Survey, and the Behavioral Risk Factor Survey Surveillance project (Broussard et al., 1991; Davis, Helgerson, & Waller, 1992).

Certain widely held values of NAs also influence research on their health. The intimate relationship between health and spirituality for traditional people may mean that NAs find it very difficult to define health or that a discussion of the topic is not socially acceptable either because one does not speak of spiritual matters to outsiders or because such talk would expose one to the risk of witchcraft or sorcery (Sobralske, 1985). The common belief in living in harmony with nature and accepting life as it comes may translate into what appears to Anglo caregivers to be passivity, fatalism, stoicism, or even self-destructive behavior. Interviews and questionnaires may conflict with NA perceptions of questioning as rude, and talking about oneself is discouraged in many NA cultures (Henderson & Primeaux, 1981).

NA family networks are often quite different from those of the larger society. The structure of NA extended families often resembles villages or multiple households with relatives along both horizontal and vertical lines, rather than the three vertical generations that mark an extended family in Anglo society. NAs may use more or different kinship terms than the general population or use the same terms differently, as when all females of the ascending generation are called "grandmother" (Henderson & Primeaux, 1981). Red Horse, Lewis, Feit, and Decker (1978) described three family lifestyle patterns (traditional, bicultural, and pan-traditional) of urban Minnesota Chippewas that seem identifiable in more recent literature from a wide variety of tribes.

Limited ability to speak, understand, or read English is a barrier to care for many NAs, particularly those of middle age and older and those from rural areas or reservations (Red Horse, Johnson, & Weiner, 1989) and a constraint on research by nonnative investigators. As language is a key indicator of biculturalism, researchers who do not assess language proficiency or preference or who exclude nonEnglish speakers may be obtaining information that is not representative of the culture.

Conducting Successful Research with Native Americans

Several classic works provide guidance for the student of NA health (Adair & Deuschle, 1970; Shore, 1989; Trimble, 1977). Their recommendations include: (a) investigators' comprehensive knowledge of the recipient culture, including its political, prestige, and clan structures, and at least a rudimentary knowledge of the language, (b) planning of research to meet the felt needs of the recipient society, (c) identification and avoidance of such negatively charged words as "research" and "experiment," (d) use of an NA advisory committee (preferably compensated) to assess the impact of the research process and possible findings on the community, (e) development of culturally sensitive instruments, (f) appreciation of the importance of acculturated individuals in transmitting new ideas to more conservative members of the tribe, (g) training of respected NAs as interviewers and lay caregivers, (h) the use of NA homes rather than clinics as primary sites for education and data collection, (i) use of the clan structure for medical records and sampling procedures, (j) investigator realism about study focus, goals, and the short-term practical application of findings (rarely accomplished in one study), (k) sharing of research findings with the community in a style meaningful to them and that will maximize relevance for program planning, (l) protection of the confidentiality of the community, as well as subject confidentiality, and (m) avoidance of press releases, which have often been "the kiss of death" for researchers in NA communities.

Reacting to the common focus on disease models that draw upon clinical populations and assume deficits in NA life, Red Horse and colleagues (1989) urged that researchers make more use of social conservation models of research, which draw on critical life circumstances of NAs to operationalize research variables. Anticipated advantages of this approach include research paradigms that capture Indian lifestyles and identify cultural strengths and research findings that guide allocation of resources for health promotion and disease prevention.

Jacobson and Booton (1991) have described their strategies for establishing a nursing research program on NA health in Oklahoma. Their report makes very clear the important facts that research with NAs requires a long-term and multifaceted effort to learn about the native culture and earn the trust and credibility of potential subjects and that investigator presence and participation in the native community not only build goodwill but result in useful insights for future research.

Instrumentation Issues in Research on NA Health

The lack of fit of existing psychological measuring instruments to native cultures and the related issues of limited proficiency in speaking or reading English have been identified as frequent problems in research on NAs (McShane, 1988; Trimble, 1977). Four research reports by nurses were located on this problem.

Cultural considerations in the use of the Piers-Harris Self-Concept Scale with 153 Montana NA children (tribe unspecified) were evaluated by Long and Hamlin (1988). The scale appeared to be an internally consistent measure of self-concept for both white and NA children, with scores for both influenced more by children's social contexts rather than by ethnicity per se. Cultural concerns about the meaning (validity) of NA scores included the possibility that the instrument's focus on individual achievement and evaluation may be inappropriate or insufficient for a culture that values one's place within the clan and tribe and in which the very meaning of "self" is unclear.

Higgins and Dicharry (1991) examined the content validity for the Brandt and Weinert Personal Resources Inventory (PRQ), Part 2, which measures respondents' perceived level of social support. Twenty-nine Navajo women judged 10 of the 25 items to be personally or culturally unacceptable. Reasons for rejection included cultural valuation of stoicism and self-reliance, cultural prohibition of discussion of personal and family problems with others, and the inappropriateness of items about work and financial problems for Navajo women whose role is defined within the family. The findings allowed preliminary definition of the concept of social support for women within this culture. This report exemplified many desirable characteristics of research with NAs, besides recognition of the need to assess the suitability of an instrument for use with another culture. Theoretical and empirical knowledge of the Navajo culture was apparent. Native interviewers were used, and translation problems were recognized and managed.

In two studies (Seideman, Haase, Primeaux, & Burns, 1992; Seideman et al., 1994) nurse investigators explored the usefulness of the Nursing Child Assessment Satellite Training instruments (NCAST) for studying parenting among NA parents. The instruments were found capable of identifying NA cultural parenting strengths such as an unhurried approach to feeding and teaching; subscale score differences between NAs and scale norms were explainable in light of known cultural values. The need to assess other caregivers within the NA family besides the biological parents was identified in order to obtain a full and culturally valid picture of children's environments, a desirable recommendation in light of the nature of the NA extended family. Strengths of these studies included the use of urban NAs, the use of both observational and verbal qualitative data collection strategies to assess the adequacy of the underlying model and the meaning of the data, the use of the home for data collection, and the assistance of NA nurses in recruiting subjects and collecting and interpreting data.

ACUTE AND CHRONIC ILLNESS

Maternal-Child and Family Health

Three studies of maternal–child and family health (defined to include coping with illness) with nurse involvement were found. The effectiveness of a prenatal consultative clinic in reducing fetal death rates among Sioux women in South Dakota was reported by Peterson et al. (1984). Strengths included a comparison group of pregnant white patients and sample sizes of over 340 per group. The approach here was essentially medical; no nursing perspective was apparent.

Although NAs have the highest incidence of sudden infant death syndrome (SIDS) in the nation, only one study of this problem was found. Bushy and Rohr (1990) surveyed NA mothers from North and South Dakota to determine social and cultural reasons for inconsistent use of home apnea monitors. Respondents completed the Norbeck Social Support Questionnaire (Norbeck, Lindsey, & Carrieri, 1981, 1983) and several questions about number of children and infant caretakers in the homes and use of the monitors. The major findings were that the most frequent sources of social support for mothers were members of the extended family, rather than their spouses, and that noncompliant mothers were younger, poorer, more likely to be single, and to have previously lost a child from SIDS than compliant mothers. Limitations of this study were the small ($N = 16$) convenience sample, lack of determination of the cultural validity of the Norbeck Scale for this population, and the likelihood of subjects' fear of reprisal for noncompliance. As the actual study was only a small part of this report, most of the cultural considerations surrounding apnea monitors presented appear to be derived from other literature sources or clinical experience.

Wuest (1991) used Canadian NA families as a theoretical sample to refine a grounded theory of family management of children's otitis media. The contrasting of NA and Caucasian management strategies revealed that NAs used harmonizing as a management strategy, whereas Caucasians attempted to direct and control the illness. Nursing implications, including the absence of an NA concept of social support, were identified. The qualitative methodology, group differences, and evidence for the conclusions were well-described. Although the sample size of seven was not unusually small for a theoretical sample, Wuest reported a 50% refusal rate.

Although no nursing studies of the mental health of NA youth were found, McShane (1988) reviewed literature from 1970 to 1985 to identify research needs in this area. His suggestions cut across several areas of this chapter. Those that are most amenable to study from a nursing perspective include studies of (a) the response of various tribal cultures to alcoholic mothers and children with fetal alcohol syndrome and the development of culturally based interventions for its prevention, (b) the definition of child abuse and neglect across differing NA and Anglo cultures, the development of culturally sensitive methods for screening for adequate treatment of children, and the development of effective strategies for preventing NA child abuse and neglect, (c) NA perceptions of normal and deviant behaviors for young children (bedwetting, thumbsucking, tantrums) and the development of identity and self-esteem, (d) the nature of depression among NA children and adolescents and on its relationship to suicide, and (e) longitudinal studies of life transitions, such as from home to school or rural to urban life, and the relative influence of socializing agents (parents, elders, peers, and teachers).

The Aging Process and Elderly Native Americans

Perhaps in keeping with their small proportion in the NA population (approximately half that of the nation as a whole), relatively little information about the quality of life and health of NA elders is available except for epidemiological data showing high rates of chronic disease.

Two reports by nurse investigators (Johnson et al., 1986, 1988) examined the mental health and life satisfaction of 58 elderly midwestern NAs (tribe unspecified) and their relationships to selected environmental factors. Six sensory factors such as hearing and vision, which facilitated socialization and decreased loneliness, were the best predictors of life satisfaction, accounting for 40% of the variance. Strengths of this research were the inclusion of literature on NA elders, recognition of the need for research on NA elders, and the use of five ethnic comparison groups. Unfortunately, the limitations recognized by the investigators (the lack of assessment of the cultural appropriateness of the instruments, lack of control for key demographic variables, and low subject: variable ratio) were significant. As no efforts were made to interpret the findings in terms of NA culture, the research did little to improve understanding of NA elderly.

One nursing study that could be categorized as either a developmental study of aging or as a study of women's health was located. Buck and Gottlieb (1991) used grounded theory to study eight Mohawk women's experiences of midlife related to concepts of time. Findings supported the developmental, rather than the decremental, model of aging. Although the need to examine midlife from the perspectives of minority cultures was a justification for the study, no description of Mohawk culture was provided and the findings were not described in relation to culture.

Weibel-Orlando (1989), a nonnurse, conducted an exemplary study of NA aging. She studied the contributions of ethnic community membership and markers of successful aging in 40 NAs, mostly of Sioux, Choctaw, and Creek origin. Successful aging was jointly defined by other members of the ethnic communities, participants' self-assessments, and the investigator's rankings of sample members. The six markers that discriminated significantly between NAs ranked high and low on successful aging could be summarized as high involvement in and altruistic service to the ethnic community. The investigator used many desirable strategies for successful research with NAs, including involvement of NAs in planning and data interpretation, inclusion of urban and rural NAs, use of a success rather than a deficit model, recognition of variability and change in the status of NA elders in their societies, and relation of findings to other conceptualizations of aging such as the disengagement model.

Research on Diabetes

As diabetes ranks high as a cause of NA morbidity and mortality, it is a frequently studied problem. More studies by nurses were found on this topic than on any other.

Lang (1985) and Tom-Orme and Hughes (1985) conducted ethnographic studies of beliefs about the cause and treatment of diabetes among the Sioux and the Northern Utes, respectively. Although a variety of indigenous and environmental etiologies for diabetes were offered, informants from both studies agreed that deviation from traditional ways was a chief source of NA vulnerability to the disease. The Ute informants evinced a fatalistic attitude toward the disease with little sense of personal responsibility for making healthful changes in their lives (Tom-Orme & Hughes, 1985). Lang (1985) reported that low compliance with prescribed diets among the Sioux appeared to be a form of political protest against Anglo interference with eating habits and an affirmation of NA identity and that 2½ years of contact with the community were needed to establish rapport and collect the data.

Tom-Orme (1984, 1988) also described development of a culturally based diabetes intervention for the Northern Utes. Although the intervention was never fully implemented because of personnel turnover and other logistic problems, it resulted in increased awareness and acceptance of diabetes as a health problem in the community and significant decreases in glycosylated hemoglobin values for the intervention group. Strengths of the research program included an assessment of the history, culture, and medical status of the Utes, extensive collaboration among tribal, state, and federal agencies, the use of both process and outcome objectives for the intervention and biophysical as well as cognitive and social measures, the use of native women as data collectors, the use of "control tribes" (unidentified in accordance with their wishes), and the development of native community health representatives into patient educators and cultural liaisons. Examples of cultural influences on the research design and process included the refusal of informants to be tape-recorded and the absence of baseline data on diabetic patients' self-care knowledge, which although attempted, was perceived as threatening by the patients. Limitations of the research reflected difficulties in conducting research within an ongoing health care program and included midstudy changes in treatment because of physician turnover and in the method of glycohemoglobin analysis, and inability to obtain pretreatment baseline data and determine reliability of data collection and coding.

In two studies nurses used stories as interventions for noninsulin dependent diabetes (NIDDM). Moody and Laurent (1984) collaborated with tribal officials and elders to adapt Seminole folktales to transmit health messages about diet, exercise, and diabetes. The stories were presented by tribal people in Seminole and English as part of a health camp for adults and were positively evaluated by campers as good ways to learn about healthy living and to teach their families. In an exemplary Canadian study, Hagey (1984) described how the Ojibway story of Nanabush, a legendary teacher and cultural model of balance, was used as a vehicle to explain the origin and nature of diabetes and to identify appropriate coping strategies while preserving the right of each individual to choose his own unique path. Based on 2 years of fieldnotes, this report provided a rich description of the Native cultures and the collaboration among a university faculty of nursing, a community center, and tribal people to plan and conduct the program. Hagey's disclosure of her professional doubts and concerns about the technique and equally frank admission that the Native judgment was superior added true humanity to this engrossing account.

MacDonald, Shah, and Campbell (1990) used Hagey's recommendations to develop a cross-cultural, cross-jurisdictional program to improve self-care of diabetes among several tribes in southern Alberta. This was the only instance identified in the literature in which a study by one nurse (Hagey, 1984) was used by another nurse (MacDonald) to plan a clinical program.

Educational and cultural challenges in designing nutrition education programs for NAs have been explored. Broussard (1989) and Hosey, Freeman, Stracqualursi, and Gohdes (1990) studied the relationships between formal education and reading levels of NAs and recommended that diabetes education materials should be prepared at the fourth to seventh grade reading level. The single concept approach to diet instruction (eat less sugar, be more active) was found to be more effective with NAs than the diet exchange concept (Stegmayer, Lovrien, Smith, Keller, & Gohdes, 1986).

Given the increase in gestational diabetes among NA women and the increased chances that their children will develop diabetes, it was surprising that no reports of interventions with NA gestational diabetics were found directed at health promotion in the children. This is definitely a needed area of research to which nurses could contribute.

Research On Cancer

Although cancer rates are significantly lower among NAs than in the general population, they are expected to increase rapidly given the increase in NA elderly and the prevalence of tobacco use among the young (DHHS, 1990). One study of cancer, conducted by a nurse, was found. At the request of an Alaskan village council, Sprott (1988) explored carcinogenic exposure histories and beliefs about the causes of cancer in seven lung cancer patients and 46 of 51 village households. The six theories of cancer causation in rank order by percentage of household agreement were drinking-water contamination and chemicals, smoking cigarettes, fallout from nuclear testing, change from traditional to Western diet, indoor air pollution from wood smoke, and outdoor air pollution and ozone layer depletion. Strengths of this study, essentially a community assessment, included support and assistance from the community council, recognition of the need to determine the community perspective before launching a cancer prevention program, and respect for the village's desire for anonymity.

AIDS Among Native Americans

Although NAs account for less than 0.07% of acquired immunodeficiency syndrome (AIDS) cases, AIDS is expected to increase rapidly in NAs, given the poverty, youth, mobility, and incidence of sexually transmitted disease and substance abuse of the population (Campbell, 1989). Claymore and Taylor (1989) reported that human immunodeficiency virus (HIV)-positive NAs may become a source of infection if they participate in tribal ceremonies involving piercing of the skin. Also, HIV-positive NAs face a greater risk of suicide and of violence from concerned members of their tribes.

In the only study located about AIDS among NAs and conducted by a nurse-author and others, Metler, Conway, and Stehr-Green (1991) compared demographic and risk characteristics of the 237 NA cases of AIDS reported to the Centers for Disease Control through 1990 with those of persons with AIDS of other racial and ethnic groups. NA AIDS was more likely to be related to intravenous drug use and to heterosexually transmitted diseases than to homosexual/bisexual contact. Almost all NA with AIDS were diagnosed in nonIndian facilities; only 9% of NA AIDS cases were initially diagnosed in an IHS facility. The authors noted that the true incidence of AIDS among NAs may be higher than recorded because of racial misclassification.

Substance Abuse Among NAs

Alcohol abuse is one of the most extensively studied NA health problems. Two reports dealing with NA substance abuse by nurses were located. Silk-

Walker, Walker, and Kivlahan (1988) reviewed studies of NA alcoholism in conjunction with an ongoing longitudinal study of substance abuse by urban NAs in the Seattle area. This report also included a critical review of the use of several common psychological instruments with NAs. Finley (1989) surveyed 2234 students from grades 6 to 12, 70 of whom were NA, to identify differences in the social networks of NA and nonNA students in regard to alcohol use. Among the many significant differences found, no NA students reported encountering social criticism of their drinking, NA parents were more likely than white parents to have supplied the alcohol, and NAs were less likely than nonNAs to cite health, others' disapproval, or another's bad experience as reasons for abstinence or moderation. Finley concluded that a school-based prevention program designed solely on health promotion would not be sufficient to impact the social network issues identified and noted that many NAs with severe drinking problems were likely to have dropped out of school before reaching the grades participating in the study. Strengths of this research included subject anonymity, efforts to assess content and construct validity of the instruments, and presence of a staff person to answer student questions and ensure independent responses to the survey. Although the use of a random sample of students was identified by the investigator as a strength, the small proportion of NA students in the sample might have been combatted by inviting all NAs to participate or at least by oversampling them.

There is a small but growing literature on NA abuse of substances other than alcohol, particularly among adolescents. In work representing a decade of funded research, Beauvais et al. (1985) reported on trends in the use of inhalants among over 10,000 NA adolescents from over 30 tribes from 1975 to 1985. They concluded that NA youth have a much higher level of exposure to inhalants than other youth (around 40%, compared to approximately 10% for a national survey in 1979), that use of inhalants has not shown the slight decline in usage noted for other drugs by NA youth, that inhalants often serve as "gateway" drugs, and that peer influence is both a major influence on inhalant use and an avenue for prevention programs. Strengths of this research were its large sample size, the timespan covered (although it resulted from combining four distinct samples rather than being truly longitudinal), and the use of a comparison group of households from another national study. The limitations of the research, such as the likelihood that the high rate of NA school dropouts resulted in underestimation of the problem and the lack of inclusion of urban NA youth, were carefully identified. This report also illustrated many of the difficulties of doing large-scale research with NAs, such as the need for extensive negotiations for permission to survey NA youth and the requirement by tribes that they not be named in publications.

Research on NA substance abuse differs from that on other NA problems in that several theoretical models (historical, physiological, socioeconomic, and psychological) of the origin of NA substance abuse exist (Lamarine, 1988). Each may be applicable to certain tribes, age groups, or settings, but their use is controversial to many NA groups.

Major gaps in the literature of NA drug use and abuse (Trimble, 1984) included an emphasis on the Navajo and other Southwest Indians and a relative lack of focus on other areas and tribes, few studies of alcohol use and abuse patterns among NA women, no quantitative studies of urban NA alcohol and drug abuse that use measures other than arrest for public drunkenness, lack of systematic investigation of alcohol and drug abuse by urban NAs despite the steadily increasing migration to cities, and little information about treatment programs that would allow other NA groups establishing new programs to learn from the successes and failures of others. Although this review is now nearly a decade old and the numbers of reports have increased, the reviewer's sense of the literature is that Trimble's assessment of the topical balance of reports is still quite accurate. The current thrust of research on abuse of alcohol and other substances (and the most likely arena for nursing involvement) concerns the development of culturally based interventions for treatment and prevention (Lamarine, 1988).

Abuse and Neglect in NA Families

Child abuse and neglect and spousal abuse in NA families have received relatively little research attention. In addition to the usual problems of studying abuse and neglect (defining it, reporting it, and gaining community cooperation), students of this problem in NA communities face the complexities of cultural variation within and across tribes, the intense reaction of NAs to the historic frequency of removal of NA children from their biological families (McShane, 1988), and the reluctance of cross-cultural researchers to refer to abuse as abuse (Lujan et al., 1989).

Lujan et al. (1989) conducted one of the very few in-depth analyses of child abuse and neglect in NA families that enjoyed Native input and cooperation. The design involved record reviews of 117 abused and neglected children, 88 parents, and 78 grandparents from 11 Pueblo tribes and 1 Apache tribe and nonreservation NAs from throughout the United States. Interviews with service providers also were used to supplement chart data, which were found to underdocument histories of alcohol abuse among caretakers. Major findings were that alcohol abuse was present in 85% of cases of neglect and 63% of cases of abuse, that abuse and neglect occurred simultaneously in 65% of the sample, that female children moved from home to home were most likely to be abused, and that multiproblem families and multigenerational histories of alcohol abuse were prominent factors in abuse and neglect. The assistance of three registered nurses was acknowledged.

In a study unusual for its comparative case study design and use of a theoretical model of community change in response to industrialization, [Blishen's (Blishen, Lockhart, Craib, & Lockhart, 1979) socioeconomic impact model for northern development], Durst (1991) studied changing attitudes toward conjugal violence in two Canadian Arctic communities. Quantitative and qualitative data about the amount of and response to conjugal violence before and after oil and gas development were collected from 51 native key informants. The findings indicated that although conjugal violence had increased (and alcohol was implicated), it was an old problem and not caused by industrialization. What had changed with industrialization was the willingness of the communities to recognize the problem and respond with community-based programs. This well-designed study demonstrated a rich knowledge of the native culture and the conditions of successful research with NAs.

HEALTH PROMOTION AND DISEASE PREVENTION

Native American Perspectives on Health and Healing

Several nurses have explored NA perspectives on health and healing through interviews and observations. Sobralske (1985) sensitively described traditional and changing health beliefs and values of the Navajo and emphasized the generally underrecognized difficulty of asking NAs to define health. (The empirical origin of the work was identified in a citation in a report by Adams and Knox, 1988.)

Adams and Knox (1988, 1993; Knox & Adams, 1991) have described ongoing research on the health beliefs and practices of the Menominee, Oneida, and Stockbridge-Munsee tribes of Wisconsin. Strengths of these reports included clear descriptions of the historic and current characteristics of the three tribes, empathy for the conflicts of belief systems encountered by NA users of health services, and recognition of individual differences in traditionality. Although the participation of an NA investigator (Adams) is ordinarily considered a strength in NA research (and appeared to be so here), the reviewer cautions from her own experience that it may also introduce demand characteristics or biasing effects from family or tribal politics.

Morse, Young, and Swartz (1991) compared Cree Indian methods of treating disease (psoriasis) with those of Western medicine. Ethnographic analysis of observations of healing rituals identified many incongruities between the two systems such as patients' passive roles in the Western system and the directive, impersonal manner of Western caregivers and illustrated the nature of holistic care and the intuitive psychology used by Native healers. A provocative description of the possible harmful ramifications of a caring/curing distinction between nursing and medicine was also present. The pairing of description and discussion for each of the five aspects of the treatment process was an excellent way to present the nature and significance of observational data.

Common strengths of these studies included the obvious respect of the investigators for NA practices and healers, use of NA homes or healing sites for data collection, and clear acknowledgment of the cultural limitations of the research, such as the possible unwillingness of subjects to share information that has religious meanings.

Health Risks and Behavior

Research on NA health risks, behavior, and knowledge as a prelude to health promotion and disease prevention in the Western sense has been hampered by the lack of information on NAs in most nationwide surveys and by the need for the Indian Health Service to devote most of its resources to acute care, but this is increasing. As no nursing studies of these matters were found, three recent studies by nonnurse investigators are presented. Data from the Behavioral Risk Factor Surveillance System (BRFSS) were judged useful for estimating behavioral risk prevalence for NAs and to monitor progress toward achievement of *Healthy People 2000* objectives (Sugarman, Warren, Oge, & Helgerson, 1992). NA risks were similar to those of whites except for smoking and overweight among women, which were higher. A strength of the design was the comparison of BRFSS data on NAs with that from household surveys and other data sets. Limitations of the BRFSS data include the low telephone coverage among NAs in many areas, the relatively small sample size of NAs (approximately 1000) for any single year of the BRFSS, and the absence of studies to validate the self-reported data in the surveys.

The most comprehensive assessment of the prevalence of overweight and obesity in NAs to date (Broussard et al., 1991) found the prevalence of overweight and obesity among NAs of all ages and both genders to be significantly higher than the US rates. The most striking findings were from NA adolescents from Arizona, where 78.3% of females from 14 to 17 years old were overweight and 51.8% were obese. Data from three national data sets were used: the National Medical Expenditure Survey (NMES) for adults ($n = 3200$), the Adolescent Health Survey and actual examinations of school children in three NA communities for school age children ($n = 12,745$), and the Centers for Disease Control Pediatric Nutrition Surveillance System for preschool children ($n = 54,775$). Limitations of the study included possible underestimation of the true prevalence of overweight and obesity in NAs, unsystematic sampling of schools and students, and no representation of adults not living on or near reservations.

Tobacco use by NAs is much higher than among Anglos (Sugarman et al., 1992) but varies markedly by region and tribe, ranging from 42% to 70% (DHHS, 1990). Davis and associates (1992) conducted the first statewide analysis of smoking rates during pregnancy among NA women. A unique feature of this study was the use of information from a state birth certificate question, "Did mother smoke at any time during pregnancy?" The reliability of birth certificate information was supported by an earlier study showing 96% to 99% agreement between birth certificate and hospital chart information about maternal smoking and marital status.

DIRECTIONS FOR FUTURE RESEARCH

As nursing research on NA health has been sparse, nursing research related to all aspects of NA health is needed. In addition to the gaps in research identified in the review, nursing research is needed on disabilities and rehabilitation needs of NAs, the effectiveness of home care for NAs in preventing deterioration of the chronically ill, NA women's health, intergenerational relations and changes in regard to health and cultural norms, the characteristics of successful NAs who do not succumb to high-risk lifestyles, and suicide prevention among NA adolescents. Nursing research should also address such conceptual and methodological issues as the testing of the applicability of existing frameworks and instruments to NA cultures and the development of culturally appropriate new frameworks and instruments.

Researchers will need to consider the balance of concerns about reliability and validity and the need for cultural and political sensitivity to the group being studied. For example, a researcher may conclude that the highest priority in a given situation is cultural sensitivity and that traditional reliability and validity are temporarily secondary. As good working relationships are established between the investigator and potential subjects, later studies may address measurement issues with more rigor.

This reviewer would urge that nursing research be multidisciplinary and that nurse investigators seek out consultants with relevant experience with NAs or avail themselves of such resources as departments of NA studies or area offices of the IHS. Nursing research on NA health should also become programmatic and move from description to intervention. NAs complain that although they have been studied extensively, they have little of practical value to show for it. Moreover, the goal of research on and with NAs should be to enable or empower them to meet their own health needs. Durst's (1991) recommendation that researchers should avoid professionalization of the problem and privatization of the solution is relevant to all students of NA health and consistent with nursing aims.

It cannot be emphasized too strongly that research on NA health should not be undertaken without the necessary grounding in knowledge of cross-cultural research, the conditions for successful research with native people, NA history and politics in general, and of the target NA group in particular. An attitude of research as usual except that the subjects happen to be NA is likely to produce, at best, misleading or useless data and, at worst, lasting harm to race relations, the research climate in native communities, and NA health care.

ACKNOWLEDGMENTS

The author wishes to acknowledge the assistance of Rob Krueger and Janis Campbell (GRAs) with literature searches and reference list preparation.

REFERENCES

Adair, J., & Deuschle, K. (1970). *The people's health: Medicine and anthropology in a Navajo community.* New York: Appleton-Century-Crofts.

Adams, L. M., & Knox, M. E. (1988). Traditional health practices: Significance for modern health care. In W. Van Horne (Ed.), *Ethnicity and health, Vol. 7* (pp. 134–155). Milwaukee, WI: University of Wisconsin System Institute on Race and Ethnicity.

Adams, L. M., & Knox, M. E. (1993). The impact of lifestyle on the health status of the Wisconsin Indians. In T. Shirer & S. Bransther (Eds.), *Native American values: Survival and renewal* (pp. 413–424). Sault Ste. Marie, MI: Lake Superior State University Press.

Arnold, R. W., Koertvelyessy, A. M., Berg, L. E., & Nutting, P. A. (1989). A research agenda for Indian health: Part II. Research in nursing. *The Provider, 14*, 134–135.

Beauvais, F., Oetting, E. R., & Edwards, R. W. (1985). Trends in the use of inhalants among American Indian adolescents. *White Cloud Journal, 3*(4), 3–11.

Blishen, B. R., Lockhart, A., Craib, P., & Lockhart, E. (1979). *Socio-economic impact model for Northern development.* Ottawa, CN: Department of Indian and Northern Affairs.

Brod, R. L., & LaDue, R. (1989). Political mobilization and conflict among western urban and reservation Indian health service programs. *American Indian Culture and Research Journal, 13*(3), 171–214.

Broussard, B. A. (1989). Nutrition education strategies for patients with limited reading skills: A Native American example. In *Nutrition education opportunities: Strategies to help patients with limited reading skills* (pp. 35–44). Columbus, OH: Ross Laboratories.

Broussard, B, Johnson, A., Himes, J. H., Story, M., Fichtner, R., Hauck, F., Bachman-Carter, K., Hayes, J., Frohlick, K., Gray, N., Valway, S., & Gohdes, G. (1991). Prevalence of obesity in American Indians and Alaska Natives. *American Journal of Clinical Nutrition, 53*, 1535–1542.

Buck, M. M., & Gottlieb, L. N. (1991). The meaning of time: Mohawk women at midlife. *Health Care for Women International, 12*, 41–50.

Bushy, A., & Rohr, K. M. (1990). The Plains Indians: Cultural considerations in the use of apnea monitors. *Neonatal Network, 8*(4), 59–66.

Campbell, G. R. (1989). The changing dimension of Native American health: A critical understanding of contemporary Native American health issues. *American Indian Culture and Research Journal, 13*(3 & 4), 1–20.

Claymore, B. J,. & Taylor, M. A. (1989). AIDS—Tribal nations face newest communicable diseases: An Aberdeen Area perspective. *American Indian Culture and Research Journal, 13*(3 & 4), 21–31.

Davis, R. L., Helgerson, S. D., & Waller, P. (1992). Smoking during pregnancy among northwest Native Americans. *Public Health Reports, 107*, 66–69.

Department of Health and Human Services. (1990). *Healthy People 2000: National health promotion and disease prevention objectives*, (DHHS Publication No. 91-50212 (PHS) 91-50212). Washington, DC: U.S. Government Printing Office.

Durst, D. (1991). Conjugal violence: Changing attitudes in two Northern Native communities. *Community Mental Health Journal, 27*, 359–373.

Finley, B. (1989). Social network differences in alcohol use and related behaviors among Indian and non-Indian students, grades 6-12. *American Indian Culture and Research Journal, 13*(3 & 4), 33–48.

Hagey, R. (1984). The phenomenon, the explanations and the responses: Metaphors surrounding diabetes in urban Canadian Indians. *Social Science and Medicine, 18*, 265–272.

Heckler, M. M. (1985). *Report of the Secretary's Task Force on Black and Minority Health*. Washington DC: U.S. Department of Health and Human Services.

Henderson, G., & Primeaux, M. (1981). *Transcultural health care*. Menlo Park, CA: Addison-Wesley.

Higgins, P. G., & Dicharry, E. K. (1991). Measurement issues addressing social support with Navajo women. *Western Journal of Nursing Research, 13*, 242–255.

Honigfeld, L. S., & Kaplan, D. W. (1987). Native American postneonatal mortality. *Pediatrics, 80*, 575–578.

Hosey, G. M., Freeman, W. P., Stracqualursi, F., & Gohdes, D. (1990). Designing and evaluating diabetes education material for American Indians. *The Diabetes Educator, 16*, 407–414.

Indian Health Service (1990). *Regional differences in Indian Health 1990*. Washington, DC: Department of Health and Human Services.

Jacobson, S. F., & Booton, D. A. (1991). Establishing a nursing research program on Native American health in Oklahoma. In A. Bushy (Ed.), *Rural Nursing, Vol. I* (pp. 348–363). Newbury Park, CA: Sage.

Johnson, F., Cook, E., Foxall, M., Kelleher, E., Kentopp, E., & Mannlein, E. (1986). Life satisfaction of the elderly American Indian. *International Journal of Nursing Studies, 23*, 164–273.

Johnson, F., Foxall, M., Kelleher, E., Kentopp, E., Mannlein, E., & Cook, E. (1988). Comparison of mental health and life satisfaction of five elderly ethnic groups. *Western Journal of Nursing Research, 10*, 613–628.

Knox, M. E., & Adams, L. M. (1991). Utilization of health care delivery systems: Traditional versus contemporary values of specific Native American tribes. In T. Shirer (Ed.), *Entering the 90's: The North American experience* (pp. 282–293). Sault Ste. Marie, MI: Lake Superior State University Press.

Lamarine, R. J. (1988). Alcohol abuse among Native Americans. *Journal of Community Health*, *13*, 143–155.

Lang, G. C. (1985). Diabetics and health care in a Sioux community. *Human Organization*, *44*, 251–260.

Long, K. A., & Hamlin, C. M. (1988). Use of The Piers-Harris Self Concept Scale with Indian children: Cultural considerations. *Nursing Research*, *37*, 42–46.

Lujan, C., DeBruyn, L. M., May, P. A., & Bird, M. E. (1989). Profile of abused and neglected American Indian children in the southwest. *Child Abuse and Neglect*, *13*, 449–461.

MacDonald, F., Shah, W. M., & Campbell, N. M. (1990). Developing the strength to fight diabetes: Assessing the education needs of Native Indians with diabetes mellitus. *Beta Release*, *14*(1), 13–16.

McShane, D. (1988). An analysis of mental health research with American Indian youth. *Journal of Adolescence*, *11*, 87–116.

Metler, R., Conway, G. A., & Stehr-Green, J. (1991). AIDs surveillance among American Indians and Alaska Natives. *American Journal of Public Health*, *81*, 1469–1471.

Moody, L. E., & Laurent, M. (1984). Promoting health through the use of storytelling. *Health Education*, *15*(1), 8–12.

Morse, J. M., Young, D. E., & Swartz, L. (1991). Cree Indian healing practices and western health care: A comparative analysis. *Social Science and Medicine*, *32*, 1361–1366.

Norbeck, J. S., Lindsey, A. M., & Carrieri, V. L. (1981). The development of an instrument to measure social support. *Nursing Research*, *30*, 264–269.

Norbeck, J. S., Lindsey, A. M., & Carrieri, V. L. (1983). Further development of the Norbeck Social Support Questionnaire: Normative data and validity testing. *Nursing Research*, *32*, 4–9.

Petersen, L. P., Leonardson, G., Wingert, R. I., Stanage, W., Gergen, J., & Gilmore, H. T. (1984). Pregnancy in Sioux Indians. *Obstetrics and Gynecology*, *64*, 519–523.

Red Horse, J., Johnson, T., & Weiner, D. (1989). Commentary: Cultural perspectives on research among American Indians. *American Indian Culture and Research Journal*, *13*(3 & 4), 267–271.

Red Horse, J. G., Lewis, R., Feit, M., & Decker, J. (1978). Family behavior of urban American Indians. *Social Casework*, *59*(2), 67–72.

Rhoades, E. R., D'Angelo, A. J., & Hurlburt, W. B. (1987). The Indian Health Service Record of Achievement. *Public Health Reports*, *102*, 356–360.

Rhoades, E. R., Reyes, L., & Buzzard, G. D. (1987). The organization of health services for Indian people. *Public Health Reports*, *102*, 352–372.

Seideman, R. Y., Haase, J., Primeaux, M., & Burns, P. (1992). Using NCAST Instruments with urban America Indians. *Western Journal of Nursing Research*, *14*, 308–321.

Seideman, R. Y, Williams, R., Burns, P., Jacobson, S. F., Weatherby, F. W., & Primeaux, M. (1994). Cultural sensitivity in assessing urban Native American parenting. *Public Health Nursing*, *11*(2), 98–103.

Shore, J. H. (1989). Transcultural research run amok or Arctic hysteria? *American Indian and Alaska Native Mental Health Research*, *2*(3), 46–50.

Silk-Walker, P., Walker, R. D., & Kivlahan, D. (1988). Alcoholism, alcohol abuse, and health in American Indians and Alaska Natives. *Behavioral health issues among American Indians and Alaska Natives* [Monograph]. *American Indian and Alaska Native Mental Health Research*, *1*, 65–93.

Sobralske, M. C. (1985). Perceptions of health: Navajo Indians. *Topics in Clinical Nursing, 7*(3), 32–39.

Sprott, J. E. (1988). Cancer causation beliefs in an Alaskan village. *Alaska Medicine, 30*(5), 155–158.

Stegmayer, P., Lovrien, F. C., Smith, M., Keller, T., & Gohdes, D. M. (1986). Designing a diabetes nutrition education program for a Native American community. *The Diabetes Educator, 15*, 64–66.

Stevenson, J. S. (1992). Review of the first decade of the *Annual Review of Nursing Research*. In J. J. Fitzpatrick, R. L. Taunton, & A. K. Jacox (Eds.), *Annual Review of Nursing Research*, Vol. 10, (pp. 11–22). New York: Springer Publishing Co.

Sugarman, J. R., Warren, C. W., Oge, L., & Helgerson, S. D. (1992). Using the Behavioral Risk Factor Surveillance System to monitor Year 2000 objectives among American Indians. *Public Health Reports, 107*, 449–456.

Tom-Orme, L. (1984). Diabetes intervention on the Uintah-Ouray reservation. In J. Uhl, (Ed.), Proceedings of the Ninth Annual Transcultural Nursing Conference (pp. 21–38). Salt Lake City, UT: Transcultural Nursing Society.

Tom-Orme, L. (1988). Chronic disease and the social matrix: A Native American diabetes intervention. *Recent Advances in Nursing, 22*, 89–109.

Tom-Orme, L., & Hughes, C. (1985). Health beliefs about diabetes mellitus in an American Indian tribe: A preliminary formulation. In M. Carter (Ed.), *Proceedings of the Seventh Annual Transcultural Nursing Conference* (pp. 126–134). Salt Lake City, UT: Transcultural Nursing Society.

Trimble, J. E. (1977). The sojourner in the American Indian community: Methodological issues and concerns. *Journal of Social Issues, 33*(4), 159–174.

Trimble, T. E. (1984). Drug abuse prevention research needs among American Indians and Alaska Natives. *White Cloud Journal, 3*(3), 22–34.

Weibel-Orlando, J. (1989). Elders and elderlies: Well-being in Indian old age. *American Indian Culture and Research Journal, 13*(3 & 4), 149–170.

Wuest, J. (1991). Harmonizing: A North American Indian approach to management of middle ear disease with transcultural nursing implications. *Journal of Transcultural Nursing, 3*(1), 5–14.

Chapter 10

Nursing Research in Korea

ELIZABETH C. CHOI
SCHOOL OF NURSING
GEORGE MASON UNIVERSITY

CONTENTS

Health Promotion
Traditional Medicine
Health Beliefs
Perceptions of Health
Gender
The Elderly
Maternal and Child Health in Korea
Social Support
Nursing Interventions
Nursing Systems
Directions for Future Research

The Republic of Korea has the most advanced nursing programs in the Orient. Nursing education programs in Korea are comparable to programs in the United States. There are eight doctoral programs in the country. The aim of this chapter is to provide insight about nursing research in the Republic of Korea by examining dissertations completed between 1982 and 1991.

Research for this overview was conducted in three parts: (a) all Korean National Library of Congress indices were reviewed for nursing dissertations; (b) three colleges were contacted for complete dissertation retrieval; and (c) future directions of Korean nursing research were assessed using data culled from an August 1991 forum sponsored by the Lambda-Alpha chapter-at-large of Sigma Theta Tau International.

By using dissertations the author was able to assess the reliability and validity of research instruments as well as the theory or framework guiding the research. Via consultation with doctoral faculty and deans, a consensus was reached that these dissertations represent the vanguard of Korean nursing research.

Out of the 77 dissertations reviewed, 75 were data-based studies; two involved issues related to curriculum. These dissertations covered a wide range of topics. In this chapter, the studies have been organized into four sections: health promotion, social support, nursing interventions, and nursing systems.

HEALTH PROMOTION

Among the studies identified for this review, 30 were descriptive and correlational and fall under the broad category of health promotion. K. B. Kim (1990), Yang (1989), and Ko (1990) identified essential health practices that contribute to health promotion for the Korean people. These practices include a strong adherence to a traditional culture that emphasizes harmony with the universe and with other human beings; beliefs in Confucianism, Taoism, or Buddhism that espouse beneficence to nature and all living things; and a continual striving for the selfless state of optimal health.

Traditional Medicine

K. S. Lee (1988) examined charcoal use as a remedy in folk medicine. The well-documented effects of charcoal, such as relief from indigestion, pain, infection, and diarrhea, were combined with the advantages of low expense, easy access, and minimal side effects.

In studies by Ro (1988) and S. S. Choi (1991), the investigators identified that an individual's state of health can be predicted by such things as how well the individual relates to people and balances both physical and spiritual needs. Although significant differences in quality of life were found between age, education, income, and religion, quality of life also was significantly correlated to an individual's current health status. Another strong correlation between quality of life and perceived health status was denoted by the psychological variables of hopefulness and spiritual well-being.

Health Beliefs

J. S. Moon (1990) developed an instrument, based on the health belief model, which measured the constructs of susceptibility, severity, benefits, barriers, and health motivation ($N = 1019$). Using discriminate analysis, the investigator was able to predict health beliefs based on such things as educational level, marital status, age, and gender. The research was well designed and implemented, using both qualitative and quantitative methods for instrument development, testing for internal consistency ($r = .8919$) and test–retest reliability ($.5716, p < .0000$). The study's weakness is that the sample population was drawn from one geographic location so that extrapolation to other areas is limited.

Perceptions of Health

In a similar study, W. J. Cho (1983) found discrepancies between perception of health behavior and actual practices ($N = 1,454$). Discrepancies between actual and desired levels of health behavior were more pronounced in preventive than in curative or developmental medicine and more salient at the individual than at the family and community levels. The study's weakness is a lack of explication on just what factors were influential and in what way.

Examining the effects of stress on ill adults ($n = 1,200$) and validating the instrument on healthy adults ($n = 1,075$), P. S. Lee (1984) found that health was affected by both positive and negative life events, although negative life events had more of an impact. Life stress was the most significant factor influencing health followed by gender, socioeconomic class, marital status, and age. There was a significant association, identified in 11 health problem areas, between the amount of stress and onset of disease. Another prospective study is needed to determine the interrelationship between stressful events and the onset of disease.

Gender

Other studies advance our understanding of how gender impacts on health (Chang, 1989; Chi, 1984). In a break from the traditional view of women in Korea, Chang studied responses to sexual satisfaction in posthysterectomy women. A major weakness is related to the study's cross-sectional design, which included posthysterectomy women from 1 to 18 months, who may differ in their response to sexual satisfaction.

The Elderly

Several studies related to health promotion in elderly populations (J. S. Kim, 1988; Y. J. Lee, 1989; M. S. Song, 1991). M. S. Song constructed a functional status prediction model for the elderly ($N = 209$) based on the ecological model framework. Three predictive constructs of elderly functional status were found: (a) personal characteristics, (b) environmental characteristics, and (c) an individual's affective response. Environmental variables had the highest indirect effect on functional status. It would seem, therefore, that decreasing depression and/or controlling environmental variables are necessary to improve the functional status of the elderly. The strength of the study is the development of the model to test multiple variables. This holistic approach goes further than other Korean researchers in this area.

In two descriptive studies, factors causing delays in seeking medical care (K. B. Shin, 1984) and sick-role behavior expectation (So, 1987) were examined. In both studies, the researchers found that subjects did not seek preventative care but waited until symptoms were bothersome to obtain health services.

Three studies used Roy's (1984) adaptation model as a conceptual framework to examine postillness adaptation (Suh, 1988), adaptation to stress (Y. K. Kim, 1990), and adaptation to fears of hospitalization (Y. I. Moon, 1991). Although further research, specifically longitudinal studies, is needed to predict what variables and factors promote health, Korean studies (Y. K. Kim, 1990; Y. I. Moon, 1991; Suh, 1988) offer new ways of viewing how philosophical and spiritual orientation may influence physical health. In contrast to Western traditions that mask health problems with instant symptom relief, traditional Korean health practices promote a lifestyle that is aligned, balanced, and in harmony with nature. In effect, Oriental philosophy promotes health and wellness even before the onset of pathology, whereas Western philosophy intervenes after the onset of illness.

Maternal and Child Health in Korea

Studies in maternal and child health generally delineate health promotion through cultural beliefs and practices that are unique to Korea. In one study, D. S. Cho (1987) identified the practice of *Taekyo*, or fetus education, in 358 pregnant Korean women and its perception among health care providers (*n* = 68). Practices had changed from traditional *Taekyo*, which emphasizes rituals and a serene environment, to a more modern version of *Taekyo*, in which the emphasis is on diet and behavior. Similarly, the perception of *Taekyo* had changed among health professionals to incorporate new concepts, such as using *Taekyo* as an opportunity for mother and fetus to interact, and for the mother-to-be to adapt to her new maternal role. The strength of this study is the incorporation of the perspectives of both mothers and health professionals.

In several studies, investigators explored different aspects of mothering with traditional Korean cultural practices. Such topics included breastfeeding (Han, 1986; T. I. Kim, 1991; Pope, 1984); maternal role expectations in handicapped and nonhandicapped groups (Storey, 1984); differences in mother–infant interaction between patients undergoing vaginal births versus cesarian births (M. Y. Cho, 1988); the development of maternal confidence over time (E. S.

Lee, 1987); an estimation of children's health using behavioral profiles (K. J. Hong, 1986); family cohesion in psychiatric and nonpsychiatric groups (S. Kim, 1983); and male adolescent mental health (Y. H. Ahn, 1988).

Finally, Y. S. Park (1991) conceptualized the transition to motherhood by primiparas in four phases: (a) the identifying phase (1 to 10 days), (b) the accepting phase (11 days to 3 weeks), (c) the shaping phase (3 to 5 weeks), and (d) the stabilizing phase (5 to 8 weeks).

Most of the studies involved early phases of motherhood. Future research should focus on multidimensional and longitudinal studies including information on multiparas, the influence of the father, and the impact of extended family on parenting and child development.

SOCIAL SUPPORT

Eleven studies used social support as a theoretical framework. Eight of these studies were experimental or quasiexperimental, and three were descriptive. Overall, the studies had smaller sample sizes and different instruments and populations. Thus, generalizations cannot be made with any certainty until further studies are conducted that can validate previous findings.

In conceptualizing social support, J. W. Park (1985) developed a tripartite scale: the need for support, the type of social support, and the social support network. Social support differed by age, gender, religion, marital status, and socioeconomic class. The study incorporated qualitative and quantitative methods in constructing and testing the instrument. In addition, it included diverse populations from different age groups, health statuses, and genders. The instrument had high internal consistency (.939) and test–retest reliability .5050 ($p < .001$). Both empirical and construct validity testing were conducted.

Several studies found increased social support from significant family members. This resulted in improved functional health by lowering anxiety (Moh, 1985), relieving stress (H. L. Ahn, 1985; H. S. Kim, 1989a; M. J. Kim, 1985), fostering better compliance (Y. H. Choi, 1984b; O. J. Park, 1985b), and decreasing depression (Y. S. Cho, 1987). C. J. Kim's study (1983) did not find any significant relationship between family visits and patient stress, however, except the expression of positive feelings by the patient after the family visit. Because this was a correlational study with no clear theoretical framework, the results of the study are weakened.

M. J. Kim (1985) studied the effects of supportive nursing care on stress relief for hospitalized patients ($N = 66$). There were significant differences in the Na excretion rate between the experimental and control groups, indicating that supportive nursing care may lower stress levels. Anxiety and uncertainty scores did not show a significant difference even though the direction was in the hypothesized way, however. A small sample size and only two measures may have contributed to these nonsignificant findings.

Oh (1990) compared social support, life events, and depression between psychiatric patients and a nonpsychiatric control group ($N = 160$). In general, the psychiatric patients experienced a higher level of life events, higher depression, and lower social support than the nonpsychiatric controls. This was a correlational study. A longitudinal prospective study needs to be undertaken to delineate the interrelationships among stress, life events, depression, and social support before the onset of psychiatric illness.

J. A. Kim (1990) conducted a study of the effects of supportive nursing care on depression, mood, and satisfaction in military patients with lower back pain ($N = 150$). The theoretical framework used was King's (1981) interpersonal theory for nursing. The experimental design for this study was a Solomon 4 group experimental design, which has the strength of observing both the main and interactive effects of intervention. Those who received supportive nursing care had lower depression levels, more positive mood changes, and increased satisfaction levels. Moreover, the effect of supportive nursing care remained the same at 1-week follow-up. This study best exemplifies a minimizing threat to external validity.

Clearer theoretical work is needed to distinguish the various conditions underlying inadequate social support in order to match interventions with the appropriate need (Norbeck, 1988). Support can be interpreted in many ways, using different models and instruments. This makes it extremely difficult to compare the overall effects of social support among various studies.

Future studies should use instruments that are standardized and that meaningfully capture social support in its multidimensionality. How does social support work in a socially dense culture that stresses the importance of family and social connectedness as a norm for social relationships? Would it be useful to compare this with the individualistic and highly mobile population of the United States, where social isolation is experienced at many levels, and professional help is more often chosen over problem-solving within the family?

Some problems of social support in Korea revolve around competing interests and differing philosophies among family members that can cause an individual to be ostracized for not conforming to family or societal values. For example, a Korean feminist would face strong pressure if she attempted to change the present patriarchal and hierarchical system and might be ostracized for doing things differently than her mother, her mother-in-law, or other members of her family. Future researchers in the Republic of Korea may need to pursue the question of when support begins to be perceived as interference.

NURSING INTERVENTIONS

Twenty studies tested nursing interventions. All were experimental in design. In three studies, investigators provided structured information to surgery patients. S. W. Lee (1982) examined the effect of such information on sleep; Doh (1983) studied its influence on rates of recovery according to modes of coping; and K. S. Kim examined the effects of preparatory information on stress reduction. There were no significant findings. The weakness of these studies may be related to the use of a single independent variable of structured information, which, by itself, may not significantly alter physiological parameters as a dependent measure.

Three studies used Orem's (1980) self-care as a conceptual framework for a nursing intervention. Kang (1985), J. S. Shin (1985), and Yu (1991) found that patients who increased their self-care experienced a higher degree of recovery. The strength of these studies is the application of the nursing model in the testing of an intervention.

In a similar vein, Y. J. Choi (1986) examined the effects of functional communication reinforcement in families of schizophrenics. The experimental group showed significant differences from the control group. Specifically, the parents in the experimental group exhibited higher recognition and understanding about the disease, the patients' mothers had lower psychopathology, and patients had a faster recovery rate. Because psychiatric illness carries a high stigma in Korean society, further studies are needed to elucidate the role of family communication in psychiatric illness.

Other experimental studies used nursing interventions that resulted in improved patient health. J. H. Lee (1984) measured the effect of sensory stimulation on the weight gain of low-birthweight infants. M. J. Kim (1987) tested a muscle-training intervention; pulmonary function was increased. H. Y. Lee (1986) found that systolic blood pressure was decreased when health contracting was used with hypertensive clients. In a study with Type II diabetic patients, June 1991 identified that jogging increased glucose and lipid metabolism and enhanced cardiopulmonary function.

Psychological studies of nursing interventions measured a variety of outcome variables. These included patient self-exploration behavior (M. S. Kim, 1984), depression (Chon, 1989), life satisfaction (Hah, 1991), and fear-reduction and cooperative behavior (J. H. Song, 1991).

J. I. Kim (1985) combined both physiological and psychological parameters. The investigator found that relaxation therapy decreased anxiety levels, blood pressure, and pulse; increased excretion of sodium and potassium r; and decreased Chlorpromazine intake.

J. S. Park (1989) studied hemodialysis patients ($n = 72$) and showed mixed results regarding the effects of relaxation techniques on stress and quality of life. Techniques included live relaxation (LR), taped relaxation (TR), and "quiet time only" (control) groups. In the LR and TR groups, pulse rate was decreased. For blood pressure, both the LR and control groups had lower systolic blood pressure. Diastolic blood pressure was lower only in the control group, however. The LR and TR groups had less psychological stress, visual analogue stress, and depression than the control group. In addition, both LR and TR groups had a higher quality of life score than the control group. The mixed results in physiological indicators need to be followed over time with a larger sample.

Three studies focused on nursing procedures that are frequently encountered in Korea. Yoo (1986) compared the relationship between preoxygenation and postoxygenation levels and changes in intracranial pressure (ICP) in patients receiving endotracheal suctioning (ETS). The group of patients receiving 100% oxygen preETS and postETS suctioning had less increase in ICP and returned to a preETS level faster than did the ICP of those with 40% oxygen. Another advantage found in providing 100% oxygen before and after ETS, is that it diminished the sustaining time of increase in ICP after the ETS.

H. S. Park (1989) assessed the nutritional status of two groups of patients ($N = 60$), one group received enteral nutritional support only and the other group received enteral feeding and passive range of motion. Despite enteral feedings, over half the subjects remained malnourished for 1 to 2 weeks after enteral support. Although not significant, those who received enteral feedings and passive range of motion did have improved nutritional status, however.

Hur (1991) compared three analgesia methods for 24-hour postoperative pain and recovery rates after gastrectomy. Except for the ability to sleep at night, there was no significant difference in physiological responses among morphine by epidural infusion, intramuscular demerol every 4 hours, and demerol as needed ($N = 30$). The epidural infusion group had a better night's sleep but also had higher urinary retention problems.

The majority of the intervention studies suffer either from one-time treatment or short duration, as well as from small sample size. In addition, they do not provide enough data for analysis, resulting in inconclusive findings. Future studies need to address not only statistical differences but meaningful differences arising from nursing interventions, and postintervention studies are necessary to monitor changes over time after treatment. Further randomization studies using larger populations are needed for the clinical application of these findings.

NURSING SYSTEMS

This section discusses 14 studies of Korean nurses and their working environments. Most of the research was exploratory and descriptive in nature. Five studies focused on the cost-effectiveness of nursing "humanpower." Categories included severity of patient need (S. S. Song, 1983), direct and indirect costs of nursing (J. H. Park, 1988), the role of the head nurse (I. S. Kim, 1988), curative services provided by community health practitioners (J. S. Kim, 1984), and home nursing care needs (S. S. Kim, 1986). These studies chart the uniqueness of nursing services in the Korean context.

Two studies concluded that strong identification of professional role behavior and role preparedness was the most influential factor governing performance level (Hahn, 1984; J. E. Park, 1984). Three studies focused on staff nurses (K. P. Hong, 1985; N. Y. Lim, 1985; S. A. Park, 1988). Lim studied circadian rhythm using Rogers' (1980) model. Changes were found in sleep patterns, increased temperature, Na excretion, and mood. No significant differences were found in circadian time. This study had a small sample ($N = 32$) so extrapolation is difficult.

K. P. Hong (1985) analyzed burnout using self-reporting of personal and job characteristics as well as social support ($N = 610$). Results indicated that hospital staff nurses in Korea perceive burnout at a considerably high level. Using a multidimensional locus of control measure, Hong found that staff nurses internality and powerful others were in inverse proportion, whereas the chance character was in direct proportion to burnout. The more job-related stress they perceived, the more they felt burnt out. Social support through social networks produced a buffering effect to burnout as well as job-related stress. This study may reflect the reality of working conditions for staff nurses in Korea, that is, a highly hierarchical and patriarchal model that does not support the individual nurse.

In a similar vein, S. A. Park (1988) studied the relationship between leadership style and nursing performance from the staff nurse's perspective ($N = 1216$). Findings showed that head nurses had a high level of traditional authority and "benevolence," and that 94% had high maturity and work competency. This finding parallels the traditional Korean style of leadership and demonstrates how Korean society may influence its nursing professionals.

The following studies examined the decision-making process in nursing practice. J. S. Choi (1984) found the nursing process was dependent on a supportive organizational environment and personal factors, such as knowledge, motivation, work satisfaction, and merit recognition. Following a physician's orders was based on a comprehensive understanding of medical personnel, physical, and patient factors (M. H. Kim, 1990). Finally, facilitative relationships by nurses fostered self-disclosure in their patients (S. O. Lee, 1988).

Yun (1991) examined the relationship among environment, organizational structure, and organizational effectiveness of public health centers ($N = 73$ health centers). The hypothesized relationship between environment and organizational structure was not supported in health centers.

A major problem in Korea's nursing system is the barrier of transforming a higher hierarchical and patriarchal social structure into a more democratic and decentralized nursing model. At present, the power base resides largely with physicians and male administrators in academia, hospitals, and public health centers. A ceiling effect exists for promotion, and many of the nursing programs remain in a subsidiary position under the control of medical schools.

Studies of the nursing system in Korea have defined unique features and contributed initial knowledge based on nursing cost, effectiveness, and leadership style that potentially can improve care for patients. Nursing systems studies are exploratory in nature and require further validation. The larger question concerning the status of nurses in Korean society remains unaddressed.

DIRECTIONS FOR FUTURE RESEARCH

As we reach the end of the twentieth century, Korean nursing research stands at a critical juncture. Although the body of knowledge developed through multiple studies has enriched the nursing field both in Korea and elsewhere, much still remains to be done. The following suggestions are based on formal reviews and open forum dialogue.

The health belief system of Korean people reflects cultural influences, integrates physical and mental health, and stresses harmony. These dissertation studies lay the groundwork for future research that will expand our current understanding of health in the context of Korean culture.

Future studies should go into greater depth and focus on more complex multidimensional and longitudinal data. The majority of dissertation studies were pilot projects.

Further validation of instruments, testing with diverse populations, and replication studies are needed before any general theory development can occur. Also, there needs to be increasing collaboration among interdisciplinary researchers.

The majority of the instruments used in Korean nursing research were translated and modified for Korean culture. It may be that instruments need to be specifically developed for Korean research. However, Meleis (1987) has stressed that authors who establish equivalency of translated instruments and tools should share this knowledge internationally, however. In addition, physiological measures need to be more precisely refined.

Overall, the main weakness of Korean nursing research lies in its lack of integration of models and nursing phenomena (Silva, 1987). This can be seen in the studies reviewed here. That is, the relationships between the conceptual model, nursing research, and nursing practice are not clearly delineated.

Given how far Korean nursing research has come despite limited resources and a long history of social constraints, the coming years should be seen as unlimited. The future will be especially bright if an effort is made among nursing communities to forge and nurture international linkages. If this comes to pass, nursing research in Korea will enter the twenty-first century with a positive contribution to make to nursing research as a whole.

ACKNOWLEDGMENTS

The author wishes to recognize Dr. Eusook Kim, Professor at Yonsei University, Dr. Susie Kim, Dean and Professor at Ewha University, and Dr. Eunok Lee, Professor at Seoul University, for their invaluable assistance with the retrieval of dissertations. The author also wishes to thank Francesca Calderone-Steichen, M.P.H., for her technical assistance and editorial advice.

REFERENCES

Ahn, H. L. (1985). *An experimental study of the effects of husband's supportive behavior reinforcement education on stress relief of primigravidas.* Unpublished doctoral dissertation, Yonsei University, Seoul, Korea.
Ahn, Y. H. (1988). *An analysis of the relationship between family adaptability and family cohesion and male adolescents mental health.* Unpublished doctoral dissertation, Yonsei University, Seoul, Korea.
Chang, S. B. (1989). *An analytic study on influencing factors for sexual satisfaction in women who have had a hysterectomy.* Unpublished doctoral dissertation, Ewha Woman's University, Seoul, Korea.
Chi, S. A. (1984). *An analysis of the relationship between middle-aged women's attitudes toward middle adulthood developmental changes and their self-reported climacteric symptoms.* Unpublished doctoral dissertation, Yonsei University, Seoul, Korea.
Cho, D. S. (1987). *A study on the taekyo behavior of women who had given birth and the health professionals perception of taekyo.* Unpublished doctoral dissertation, Yonsei University, Seoul, Korea.
Cho, M. Y. (1988). *Primiparas' perceptions of their delivery experience and their maternal-infant interaction.* Unpublished doctoral dissertation, Ewha Woman's University, Seoul, Korea.
Cho, W. J. (1983). *An empirical study on Korean adults' perception of their health behavior.* Unpublished doctoral dissertation, Yonsei University, Seoul, Korea.
Cho, Y. S. (1987). *The effects of the husband's emotional support on the prevention of postpartum depression: Using an experimental teaching intervention.* Unpublished doctoral dissertation, Ewha Woman's University, Seoul, Korea.
Choi, J. S. (1984). *A study of the factors having affect on the planned change of nursing practice.* Unpublished doctoral dissertation, Yonsei University, Seoul, Korea.
Choi, S. S. (1991). *A correlational study on spiritual well-being, hope and perceived health status of urban adults.* Unpublished doctoral dissertation, Yonsei University, Seoul, Korea.

Choi, Y. H. (1984). *An experimental study of the effects of supportive nursing intervention on family support behavior.* Unpublished doctoral dissertation, Yonsei University, Seoul, Korea.

Choi, Y. J. (1986). *A study of the effects that family approach through reinforcement of functional communication affects schizophrenics.* Unpublished doctoral dissertation, Ewha Woman's University, Seoul, Korea.

Chon, S. J. (1989). *Reminiscence: Content analysis and its nursing implication.* Unpublished doctoral dissertation, Yonsei University, Seoul, Korea.

Doh, B. N. (1983). *Effects of structured preoperative patients teaching on rate of recovery according to modes of coping.* Unpublished doctoral dissertation, Yonsei University, Seoul, Korea.

Hah, Y. S. (1991). *The effect of a group reminiscence on the psychological well-being of the elderly.* Unpublished doctoral dissertation, Seoul National University, Seoul, Korea.

Hahn, Y. B. (1984). *An analysis of nurses' socialization process in relation with perceptual orientation, role behavior characteristics and self actualization.* Unpublished doctoral dissertation, Yonsei University, Seoul, Korea.

Han, K. J. (1986). *A phenomenological study on mother-infant interacting behavior patterns related to newborn infant feeding in Korea.* Unpublished doctoral dissertation, Ewha Woman's University, Seoul, Korea.

Hong, K. J. (1986). *A study on the development of behavior profile for the elementary school children in Korea.* Unpublished doctoral dissertation, Ewha Woman's University, Seoul, Korea.

Hong, K. P. (1985). *An analytic study on burnout in relation with personal and job-related characteristics and social support.* Unpublished doctoral dissertation, Yonsei University, Seoul, Korea.

Hur, H. K. (1991). *The effect of three analgesic administration methods on postoperative pain and recovery rate after gastrectomy.* Unpublished doctoral dissertation, Yonsei University, Seoul, Korea.

Jun, J. Y. (1991). *The effects of programmed jogging on metabolism and cardiopulmonary function in Type II diabetic patients.* Unpublished doctoral dissertation, Yonsei University, Seoul, Korea.

Kang, H. S. (1985). *An experimental study of the effects of reinforcement education for rehabilitation on hemiplegia patients' self-care activities.* Unpublished doctoral dissertation, Yonsei University, Seoul, Korea.

Kim, C. J. (1983). *An empirical study on patient stress and family visiting.* Unpublished doctoral dissertation, Yonsei University, Seoul, Korea.

Kim, H. S. (1989). *The effects of an emotional and informational support group on the stress of mother with a chronically ill child.* Unpublished doctoral dissertation, Yonsei University, Seoul, Korea.

Kim, I. S. (1988). *Analysis of the work of the head nurse and a work model for the head nurse in university hospitals in Korea.* Unpublished doctoral dissertation, Yonsei University, Seoul, Korea.

Kim, J. A. (1990). *The effect of supportive nursing care on depression, mood and satisfaction in military patients with low back pain.* Unpublished doctoral dissertation, The Graduate School of Yonsei University, Seoul, Korea.

Kim, J. I. (1985). *A study of the effects of relaxation therapy upon the anxiety level of psychiatric inpatients.* Unpublished doctoral dissertation, Yonsei University, Seoul, Korea.

Kim, J. S. (1984). *Analytical study performance of the community health practitioner in primary health care in Korea.* Unpublished doctoral dissertation, Yonsei University, Seoul, Korea.

Kim, J. S. (1988). *A study of social activities and ego integrity of the aged.* Unpublished doctoral dissertation, Ewha Woman's University, Seoul, Korea.

Kim, K. B. (1990). *Ethnoscientific approach of health practice in Korea.* Unpublished doctoral dissertation, Ewha Woman's University, Seoul, Korea.

Kim, K. S. (1989). *The effect of preparatory information on stress reduction in patients undergoing cardiac catheterization.* Unpublished doctoral dissertation, Seoul National University, Seoul, Korea.

Kim, M. H. (1990). *Clinical analysis of nurse's decision in performing doctor's orders.* Unpublished doctoral dissertation, Yonsei University, Seoul, Korea.

Kim, M. J. (1985). *An experimental study of the effects of supportive nursing care on stress relief for hospitalized patients.* Unpublished doctoral dissertation, Yonsei University, Seoul, Korea.

Kim, M. J. (1987). *A clinical study on the effects of respiratory muscle training in patients with chronic obstructive pulmonary disease.* Unpublished doctoral dissertation, Yonsei University, Seoul, Korea.

Kim, M. S. (1984). *An experimental study of the effects of facilitative relationship training on nurse's helping behavior and patient's self-exploration behavior.* Unpublished doctoral dissertation, Ewha Woman's University, Seoul, Korea.

Kim, S. (1983). *An analysis of the relationship between family incongruence about family environment and the occurrence of psychiatric illness.* Unpublished doctoral dissertation, Yonsei University, Seoul, Korea.

Kim, S. S. (1986). *An exploratory study of home nursing care needs and the implementation of home nursing care.* Unpublished doctoral dissertation, Yonsei University, Seoul, Korea.

Kim, T. I. (1991). *Primiparous mothers' perceptions of their infants, child-rearing attitudes and mother-infant interactions during early feeding experiences.* Unpublished doctoral dissertation, Ewha Woman's University, Seoul, Korea.

Kim, Y. K. (1990). *An analysis on the pathway between chronic renal failure patients' stress and adaptation.* Unpublished doctoral dissertation, Ewha Woman's University, Seoul, Korea.

King, I. M. (1981). *A theory for nursing: Systems, concepts, process.* New York: Wiley.

Ko, S. H. (1990). *Korean concepts of mental health: Toward the development of nursing theory.* Unpublished doctoral dissertation, Ewha Woman's University, Seoul, Korea.

Lee, E. S. (1987). *A study of the relationship between the primiparous' self-confidence on the maternal role and the sensitivity in mother-infant interactions on feeding context.* Unpublished doctoral dissertation, Ewha Woman's University, Seoul, Korea.

Lee, H. Y. (1986). *A study of the effects of health contracting on compliance with health behaviors in clients with hypertension.* Unpublished doctoral dissertation, Yonsei University, Seoul, Korea.

Lee, J. H. (1984). *An experimental study of the effects of sensory stimulation on the low birth weight infant's early growth and development.* Unpublished doctoral dissertation, Ewha Woman's University, Seoul, Korea.

Lee, K. S. (1988). *A study on the use of charcoal as a folk medicine.* Unpublished doctoral dissertation, Yonsei University, Seoul, Korea.

Lee, P. S. (1984). *A methodological research on the measurement of stress related to life events.* Unpublished doctoral dissertation, Yonsei University, Seoul, Korea.

Lee, S. O. (1988). *A study on the facilitative relationships of patient's nurse and patient's self-disclosure/response in early stage of admission.* Unpublished doctoral dissertation, Yonsei University, Seoul, Korea.

Lee, S. W. (1982). *The effect of structured information on the sleep amount of patients undergoing open heart surgery.* Unpublished doctoral dissertation, Yonsei University, Seoul, Korea.

Lee, Y. J. (1989). *A study on the development of health assessment tool in Korean elderly.* Unpublished doctoral dissertation, Ewha Woman's University, Seoul, Korea.

Lim, N. Y. (1985). *The effect of shift rotation on the circadian rhythm.* Unpublished doctoral dissertation, Yonsei University, Seoul, Korea.

Meleis, A. I. (1987). International nursing research. In J. J. Fitzpatrick & R. L. Taunton (Eds.), *Annual review of nursing research*, Vol. 5 (pp. 205–227). New York: Springer Publishing Co.

Moh, K. B. (1985). *An analysis of the relationship between social support and anxiety which adult patients perceive.* Unpublished doctoral dissertation, Ewha Woman's University, Seoul, Korea.

Moon, J. S. (1990). *A study of instrument development for health belief of Korean adults.* Unpublished doctoral dissertation, Yonsei University, Seoul, Korea.

Moon, Y. I. (1991). *Identification and measurement of hospital-related fears in hospitalized school-aged children.* Unpublished doctoral dissertation, Ewha Woman's University, Seoul, Korea.

Norbeck, J. S. (1988). Social support. In J. J. Fitzpatrick, R. L. Taunton, & J. A. Benoliel (Eds.), *Annual review of nursing research*, Volume 6 (pp. 85–109). New York: Springer Publishing.

Oh, K. O. (1990). *A comparative study on relationship of social support, life events, and depression between psychiatric patients and normal subjects.* Unpublished doctoral dissertation, Yonsei University, Seoul, Korea.

Orem, D. E. (1980). *Nursing: Concepts of practice* (2nd ed.). New York: McGraw-Hill.

Park, H. S. (1989). *Assessment of the nutritional deficiency of patients on enteral nutritional support.* Unpublished doctoral dissertation, Ewha Woman's University, Seoul, Korea.

Park, J. E. (1984). *The relationship of role expectation, role preparedness and role behavior of nurse practitioner.* Unpublished doctoral dissertation, Yonsei University, Seoul, Korea.

Park, J. H. (1988). *A study on the determination of nursing cost for hospitalization based on the Korean diagnosis-related groups (K-DRGs) in Korea.* Unpublished doctoral dissertation, Ewha Woman's University, Seoul, Korea.

Park, J. S. (1989). *The effect of relaxation technique on stress and quality of life of hemodialysis patients.* Unpublished doctoral dissertation, Yonsei University, Seoul, Korea.

Park, J. W. (1985). *A study to develop a scale of social support.* Unpublished doctoral dissertation, Yonsei University, Seoul, Korea.

Park, O. J. (1985). *The effect of social support on compliance with sick-role behavior in diabetic patients.* Unpublished doctoral dissertation, Yonsei University, Seoul, Korea.

Park, S. A. (1988). *An exploratory study on the relationship between leadership style and performance in Korean nursing units.* Unpublished doctoral dissertation, Seoul National University, Seoul, Korea.

Park, Y. S. (1991). *Transition to motherhood of primiparas in postpartum period.* Unpublished doctoral dissertation, Seoul National University, Seoul, Korea.

Pope, M. A. (1984). *The influence of the traditional Korean childbearing culture on breast feeding.* Unpublished doctoral dissertation, Yonsei University, Seoul, Korea.

Ro, Y. J. (1988). *An analytical study of the quality of life of the middle-aged in Seoul.* Unpublished doctoral dissertation, Yonsei University, Seoul, Korea.

Rogers, M. E. (1980). *Nursing: A science of unitary human beings.* In J. P. Riehl & C. Roy (Eds.), *Conceptual models for nursing practice,* 2nd ed. (pp. 329–337). New York: Appleton-Century-Crofts.

Roy, C. (1984). *Introduction to nursing: An adaptation model.* (2nd ed.) Englewood Cliffs, NJ: Prentice-Hall.

Shin, J. S. (1985). *The effects of the range on motion exercise on self-care activities and depression.* Unpublished doctoral dissertation, Yonsei University, Seoul, Korea.

Shin, K. B. (1984). *Determinants of delay in seeking medical care in cancer patients.* Unpublished doctoral dissertation, Ewha Woman's University, Seoul, Korea.

Silva, M. C. (1987). Conceptual models of nursing. In J. J. Fitzpatrick & R. L. Taunton (Eds.), *Annual review of nursing research,* Volume 5 (pp. 229–246). New York: Springer Publishing Co.

So, H. Y. (1987). *An exploratory study of the sick role of the Korean: About the normative expectation of role exemption of normal population.* Unpublished doctoral dissertation, Ewha Woman's University, Seoul, Korea.

Song, J. H. (1991). *The effect of supportive care filmed modeling on the fear-reduction of hospitalized children facing needle-related procedures.* Unpublished doctoral dissertation, Ewha Woman's University, Seoul, Korea.

Song, M. S. (1991). *Construction of a functional status prediction model for the elderly.* Unpublished doctoral dissertation, Seoul National University, Seoul, Korea.

Song, S. S. (1983). *Estimation of optimum hospital nursing manpower by patient classification system.* Unpublished doctoral dissertation, Ewha Woman's University, Seoul, Korea.

Storey, M. (1984). *An analysis of factors influencing maternal role acquisition in mothers of handicapped children, focusing on a comparison with mothers of non-handicapped children.* Unpublished doctoral dissertation, Yonsei University, Seoul, Korea.

Suh, M. J. (1988). *The study of factors influencing the state of adaptation of the hemiplegic patients.* Unpublished doctoral dissertation, Seoul National University, Seoul, Korea.

Yang, S. O. (1989). *Korean concepts of health.* Unpublished doctoral dissertation, Ewha Woman's University, Seoul, Korea.

Yoo, J. S. (1986). *A clinical study of the relationship between pre- and post-oxygenation amounts and changes in intracranial pressure in patients receiving endotracheal suctioning.* Unpublished doctoral dissertation, Ewha Woman's University, Seoul, Korea.

Yu, S. J. (1991). *Effect of discharge education on the self-care performance of schizophrenics.* Unpublished doctoral dissertation, Seoul National University, Seoul, Korea.

Yun, S. N. (1991). *A study on relationships between environment, organizational structure, and organizational effectiveness of public health centers in Korea.* Unpublished doctoral dissertation, Seoul National University, Seoul, Korea.

Index

Contents of Previous Volumes

VOLUME III

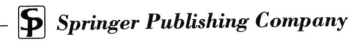
Springer Publishing Company

PREPARING NURSING RESEARCH FOR THE 21ST CENTURY
Evolution, Methodologies, Challenges

Faye G. Abdellah, EdD, ScD, RN, FAAN
Eugene Levine, PhD

with a Foreword by **C. Everett Koop**, MD, ScD

This book offers an authoritative review and critique of the state of nursing research, and a forecast of its future directions. It describes the most important methodologies currently in use and those that will be important in the future in a clear and jargon-free format.

"The purpose of this book is to share with readers our assessment of the past and present status of nursing research in order to project its future... We raise a number of important questions...and attempt to provide answers....What has nursing research achieved in the past 40 years?... What methodologies have been used in nursing research and which are the most promising for future studies? Are patients/clients better off because of the results of nursing research?... We have attempted to provide clear, concise descriptions and explanations of topics that are often confusing, controversial, or even mysterious.... Rather than another "how to do it" orientation, we take a more critical and analytical approach, emphasizing "why to do it...." —**From the Preface**

1994   288pp   0-8261-8440-5   hardcover

536 Broadway, New York, NY 10012-3955 • (212) 431-4370 • Fax (212) 941-7842

ORDER FORM

Save 10% on Volume 13 with this coupon.

___ Check here to order the ANNUAL REVIEW OF NURSING RESEARCH, Volume 13, 1995 at a 10% discount. You will receive an invoice requesting prepayment.

Save 10% on all future volumes with a continuation order.

___ Check here to place your continuation order for the ANNUAL REVIEW OF NURSING RESEARCH. You will receive a pre-payment invoice with a 10% discount upon publication of each new volume, beginning with Volume 13, 1995. You may pay for prompt shipment or cancel with no obligation.

Name _____

Institution _____

Address _____

City/State/Zip _____

Examination copies for possible adoption are available to instructors "on approval" only. Write on institutional letterhead, noting course, level, present text, and expected enrollment (include $3.50 for postage and handling). Prices slightly higher overseas. Prices subject to change.

Mail this coupon to:
SPRINGER PUBLISHING COMPANY
536 Broadway, New York, N.Y. 10012